Wolfgang Ecker

Medical Devices and IVDs

Fit for the new EU-Regulations

Your complete seminar
for project, study and job

Wolfgang Ecker

Medical Devices and IVDs
Fit for the new EU-Regulations

Your complete seminar

for project, study and job

Despite careful processing, all information in this work is provided without guarantee. Liability of the author and the publisher is excluded.

Bibliografische Information der Deutschen Nationalbibliothek:

Die Deutsche Nationalbibliothek verzeichnet diese Publikation in der Deutschen Nationalbibliografie; detaillierte bibliografische Daten sind im Internet über http://dnb.dnb.de abrufbar.

© 4th edition, April 2022, Dr. Wolfgang Ecker

Herstellung und Verlag:

BoD – Books on Demand, Norderstedt

ISBN: 9783754385395

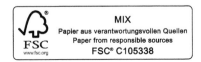

Contents

Preface

With this book, you'll get a really complete seminar for the new Regulations of medical devices/IVDs in the EU, ready at hand, at any time.
The book will give you a quick, reliable overview of this new, often perceived as rather difficult EU regulatory environment.
You will save yourself quite a lot of money and energy of countless seminars, whether in presence or, often no less strenuous, online via Zoom or MS Teams etc.
All important aspects are thoroughly prepared. Therefore, you can go into depth with each partial seminar/chapter if required.
And when it comes to the final detail, the many target-oriented references to the new EU interpretative documents and standards will help you. You will be able to act on an equal footing with authorities, notified bodies, other economic actors or the staff of research or health institutions and always have a clear direction in front of your eyes.
Use this complete seminar for the benefit of our patients, whether you work in relevant projects, in your studies, in small or larger companies, in education, in consulting or in research and health care institutions!

In 2017, after more than four years of legal work, the European legislator presented a comprehensive revision of the legislation for medical devices and in vitro diagnostics. The aim was to create a reliable legal basis, now directly applicable EU law[1], for a very dynamically growing industrial healthcare sector. This sector is characterized by rapid innovation, start-ups, spin-offs, small and medium-sized enterprises and the need for continuous training and further education, more than almost any other sector. In addition to the technical, biological and clinical sciences, regulatory know-how here plays a special role in knowledge management for development and success. In the training and further education of young people and employees, which are crucial for maintenance and further development of research and business sites, the know-how necessary for regulatory compliance must therefore not be lacking alongside the other factors! Countless failures and malinvestments are due to the lack of regulatory compliance in SMEs and

---

[1] 2 Regulations: MDR: Medical Device Regulation (EU) 2017/745 and IVDR: In vitro Diagnostic Regulation (EU) 2017/746

11

start-ups (usually without their own regulatory affairs department). How many research projects have dragged a prototype across the finish line of the project without even thinking about possible market access. They have thus wasted the most valuable time or even missed the connection to the market! The new EU regulations on medical devices and IVDs prescribe a clear reorientation for the many small manufacturers, because regulatory compliance is now very explicitly part of the obligatory quality management system (QMS) with its more clearly defined life cycle processes and is to become effective across portfolios. **A clear benefit of MDR and IVDR: The clear regulatory pathway under the QMS with close take-up of the crucial life-cycle processes and steps!** Once mentally and organisationally incorporated, this will make the life of all manufacturers and other stakeholders much more easier.

The starting points of the new regulations were above all:
- the European commitment to better anchor jointly developed global GHTF/IMDRF guidelines in the EU legal system (e.g. UDI; technical documentation; classification, conformity assessment and performance evaluation of IVDs) in order to facilitate global market access for European companies,
- Desire for more legal clarity through the transfer of non-legally-binding, especially MEDDEV, guidelines content into the legal framework (especially vigilance, clinical evaluation),
- Political will for increased transparency of the system for all stakeholders and the public through a new European database EUDAMED, combined with better product identification and traceability by the UDI system (Unique Device Identifier),
- the political will to raise level and harmonisation of the EU conformity assessment for medical devices and IVDs and of the performance of notified bodies. Particularly in the case of implants and other high-risk products, perceived challenges to the credibility of the European system had to be tackled to assure patients are treated with well assessed, safe and effective MDs/IVDs. The so-called PIP scandal was only a bold marker; the European legislator had also identified problems with other implants and high-risk products, some of which were permitted in the EU, but had failed in other jurisdictions or concerning devices already marketed elsewhere, with no critical reassurance by EU NBs. HTA assessments, being more frequently asked now by European health care

providers for reimbursement decisions, are often identifying insufficient clinical evidence provided for licensed high-risk medical devices. The health care providers wanted a more seamless transition between markets and health care systems. The legislative aims were therefore inter alia:

- significant improvement[2] of clinical evaluation of medical devices and performance evaluation of IVDs; creation of a suitable clinical expert infrastructure and of specific, more clinically oriented guidelines as in the US and in the pharmaceutical sector; creation of suitable instruments to analyse and guarantee the safety, effectiveness and performance of products over longer periods of time ('real world data' or 'post launch evidence generation', e.g. as systematic evaluations of suitable implant registries, long-term studies, evaluation of biobanks, evaluation of (valid) Big Data etc., supplemented by PMS, PMCF, PMPF[3] and risk management as strong life cycle processes);
- create a more homogeneous clinical research landscape in the EU on pharmaceuticals, medical devices and IVDs, especially for combination studies,
- the adaptation of the sector to the EU's "New Legislative Framework (NLF)" in the regulation of products, including explicit 'rules of the game' for all economic operators, in particular the manufacturer. Important: the manufacturer has to follow a clearer regulatory orientation in the obligatory QMS (see Fig. 5 and 6 and Tab. 1 as a general orientation). (Joint) market surveillance by Competent Authorities has been improved accordingly;
- Desire for better future agility of the system, e.g. in order to adequately respond to the increasing importance of companion diagnostics in personalized medicine and to medical genetic tests; as well as to the increasing importance of software in the medical devices and IVD sector, including medical device apps.

The result is a comprehensive and complex legal framework that needs to be studied carefully.

---

[2] Along and beyond MEDDEV 2.7.1 rev 4
[3] See list of Abbreviations!

In addition to the many legal changes, there is still a crisis concerning notified bodies (NBs; "European Conformity Assessment Bodies") under the European system; while past problems of quality are now being solved, there is still a problem of quantity of available NBs, esp. for the IVDR.

Although the NB market is responding with an enormous 'upgrade', it is an exciting question whether sufficient and rapid renewal of the Notified Bodies, who also still have to 'grapple' with the new legislation and reengineer themselves, can guarantee a smooth transition into the certification world of the new regulations.

Change and rapid adaptations will therefore continue to be the proverbial constant in the coming years.

What is needed now is a reliable 'GPS' based on solid basic knowledge of the new regulations and clear expectations that the regulatory, interpretative and normative environment will continue to evolve in the near future. But as always: manufacturers will have to do their thing in a targeted and prudent manner. Despite the larger size of the MDR/IVDR compared to the previous Directives: There is a lot of old wine in new wineskins! Do not enter in a panic mode! This is also true for the IVDR under the conditions of the COVID-19 crisis. Prolonged transition times through the recent amendment regulation (EU) 2022/112 of IVDR should allow for a more smooth transition, after the MD sector now also in the IVD sector and will hopefully lead to the build-up of a proper network of NBs in both sectors. A lot of things will make life of manufacturers easier now:

For example, the contents of technical documentation (in Annexes II and III) are clearly defined for the first time, there are clear legal provisions for the new labelling and instructions for use; the life cycle processes (such as clinical evaluation of MD, performance evaluation of IVD, risk management, PMS, vigilance, registration obligations, regulatory requirements under the QMS) are much more precise and often derived from previous guidelines.

See the present vademecum as a compact training course designed to provide important assistance in this regard. It is intended

1. to provide a quick and reliable overview of the new regulatory system and its components and important types of documents (see esp. Fig. 1 to 7 and Tab. 2 as a roadmap and "GPS"), and

2. to elaborate on the essential components and processes of the new regulatory system along the life cycle of the products, so that the own study of

the legal texts, which can never be dispensed with, may succeed all the easier, combined with the subsequent implementation in practice. It was also important here to provide a clear overview of the many interpretative documents which can provide valuable assistance, and which will be successively adapted to the regulations in the coming years.

The content of this compact regulatory course is derived from 2 main sources:

- the author's experience out of many years of relevant professional activity in the Austrian Health Ministry, at EU level as a co worker in many EU working groups of the sector (including chairmanship of the EU's Working Group 'Clinical Investigation and Evaluation [CIE]'), as a co-negotiator of the new regulations in Council and at the level of GHTF as one of the European representatives in Study Group 5 on Clinical Evidence, and
- the lecture activities at universities of applied sciences for medical technology and biomedical engineering, seminars for actors in business and health care, lectures for medical technology clusters as well as courses for clinical investigators.

May the course provide valuable orientation and help for the education and training of biomedical and medical technology professionals, the health professions and the training and further education of employees in companies and health care facilities, as well as for research, development and consulting projects in medical technology, biomedical and clinical engineering and related areas.

Preface to the 4th edition:
The new legal framework has in the meantime been amended several times by corrigenda and by amendments of the Medical Device Regulation (MDR) and now also the In-vitro Diagnostics Regulation (IVDR), with new transition provisions and time limits, partly to accommodate for the COVID crisis.
Since the last edition of this book, also a lot of very important interpretative guidance by the EU Medical Device Coordination Group (MDCG) has accumulated and has now to be considered in the new edition.
Vienna, February 202

Legal note:

The authentic versions of the relevant legal acts, including their preambles, are those published in the Official Journal of the European Union and available in EUR-Lex. The information and views contained in this book are those of the author and do not represent the official opinion of the European Communities or of EU Member States. Despite careful processing, all information in this work is provided without guarantee; liability on the part of the author or the publisher is excluded.

It is therefore essential to study the authentic legal texts and the interpretative guidelines available; it is advisable to use (authentic) consolidated versions of the legal texts. In case of doubt, it is often advisable to consult the competent authorities or the European Commission. The legally binding interpretation of the EU legal texts is reserved to the European Court of Justice.

Should this publication contain links to third-party websites, the author accepts no liability for their contents, as he does not adopt them as his own, but merely refers to their status at the time of initial publication.

Gender:

For reasons of easier legibility, the masculine form is predominantly used for designations of persons and functions. It also applies in the female form, of course.

Acknowledgements:

My thanks go to my national, European and international colleagues in the field of medical devices for their decades of pleasant and exciting cooperation and in particular to DI Dr Martin Renhardt and Dr Reinhard Berger from the Austrian authorities, as well as to my long-standing German colleague Dr Gert Schorn, who introduced me thoroughly to the "EU system" at a young age and to whom I have enjoyed a pleasant friendship ever since.

I am also grateful for valuable input from Elisabeth Mertl for critical reading, esp. on the preclinical evaluation of MDs, Martina and Martin for critical reading of various chapters, Andreas Aichinger, Michael Ring and Prof. Gerold Labek for fruitful discussion on important practical issues.

My special thanks also go to my wife Sigrid for lecturing and for her constant efforts to achieve a reasonable work-life balance and to Felix Ecker for helping with the graphic design.

Photo credits, image sources (cover, photos taken by W.E. with permission):

University of Applied Sciences Linz – Medical Technology, (spinal column X-ray-phantom, laboratory equipment, examination microscope); special thanks to Prof. DI Dr Martin Zauner, Msc, Dean of the Faculty of Medical Technology and Applied Social Sciences of the FH OOE and his staff;

Sozialmedizinisches Zentrum Ost, Danube Hospital, Technical Directorate, (NMR, Mammography-US) Special thanks to Mr. TOAR Ing. Manfred Führer, Technical Director, and his staff.

I would like to thank Felix Ecker for the graphic composition.

Chapter 1. Overview of the New Regulatory System for Medical Devices and In Vitro Diagnostics in the EU

Let us first take a look at the transition from the current system of EU directives to the new EU regulations for medical devices and IVDs (chapter 1.1.). Then we look at the construction principles of the new regulatory system (chapter 1.2.) and finally further to its central concepts for EU internal market access (chapter 1.3.). The most important documents of the new (and partly old) regulatory system are systematically discussed (section 1.4.). We then need a short regulatory compliance walkthrough along the product life cycle, from product development, preparation for market access, conformity assessment to the obligations when keeping the product on the EU market (section 1.5.). This fundamental orientation is concluded by the transition regime from the old directives to the new regulations with relevant time frames (section 1.6.) which have been adapted recently by the EU legislators to address urgent issues of the covid-19 crisis.

1.1. Transition from Directives to Regulations

In 2017, the EU legislator transformed the previous regulatory system for medical devices, consisting of 3 EU directives and their national implementations, into a new system of 2 EU regulations. as now directly applicable EU law (see Fig. 1):

Regulation (EU) 2017/745 on medical devices (MDR)[4], and
Regulation (EU) 2017/746 on in vitro diagnostic medical devices (IVDR)[5].
Both regulations were developed in parallel and each consist of (see Fig.2+3)

- **Recitals**, i.e. intentions and objectives of the EU legislator which can be used as an aid to interpretation in the event of legal uncertainties,
- the **Chapters and their Articles**, with the core of both legal texts, and
- the **Annexes**, the binding, more technically oriented legal text, which supplement the chapters (for example Annex I on General Safety and

---

[4] MDR consol text 24-04-2020: https://eur-lex.europa.eu/legal-content/EN/TXT/?uri=CELEX:02017R0745-20200424
[5] IVDR consol text 28-01-2022: https://eur-lex.europa.eu/legal-content/EN/TXT/HTML/?uri=CELEX:02017R0746-20220128&from=DE

Performance Requirements [GSPR; Annex II and III on technical documentation or Annexes IX to XI on conformity assessment modules [= modules of "European Premarket Approval"]).

The MDR/IVDR entered into force at EU level on 25 May 2017; the date of application for the MDR has been – after an amendment of the MDR - 26 May 2021 (4-year transitional period); for the IVDR, the date of application will be 26 May 2022 (5-year transitional period). For the more special transition periods and regimes, see chapter 1.6. in this book.

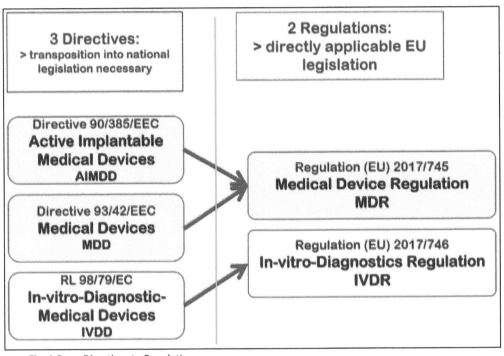

Fig. 1 From Directives to Regulations

Fig. 2 MDR: Structure and Content Overview

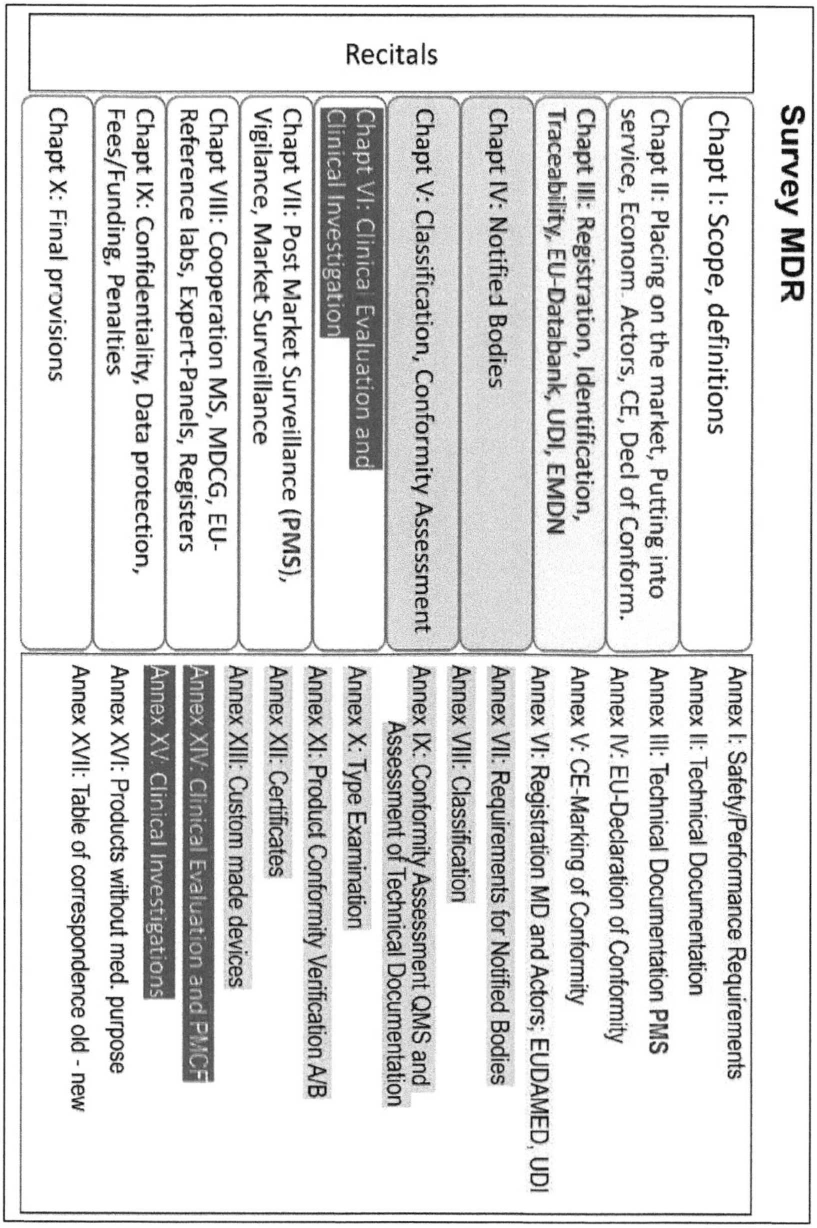

Survey MDR

Recitals

Chapt I: Scope, definitions	Annex I: Safety/Performance Requirements
	Annex II: Technical Documentation
Chapt II: Placing on the market, Putting into service, Econom. Actors, CE, Decl of Conform.	Annex III: Technical Documentation **PMS**
	Annex IV: EU-Declaration of Conformity
Chapt III: Registration, Identification, Traceability, EU-Databank, UDI, EMDN	Annex V: CE-Marking of Conformity
	Annex VI: Registration MD and Actors; EUDAMED, UDI
Chapt IV: Notified Bodies	Annex VII: Requirements for Notified Bodies
	Annex VIII: Classification
Chapt V: Classification, Conformity Assessment	Annex IX: Conformity Assessment QMS and Assessment of Technical Documentation
	Annex X: Type Examination
Chapt VI: Clinical Evaluation and Clinical Investigation	Annex XI: Product Conformity Verification A/B
	Annex XII: Certificates
Chapt VII: Post Market Surveillance (PMS), Vigilance, Market Surveillance	Annex XIII: Custom made devices
	Annex XIV: Clinical Evaluation and PMCF
Chapt VIII: Cooperation MS, MDCG, EU-Reference labs, Expert-Panels, Registers	Annex XV: Clinical Investigations
	Annex XVI: Products without med. purpose
Chapt IX: Confidentiality, Data protection, Fees/Funding, Penalties	Annex XVII: Table of correspondence old - new
Chapt X: Final provisions	

Fig. 3 IVDR: Structure and Content Overview

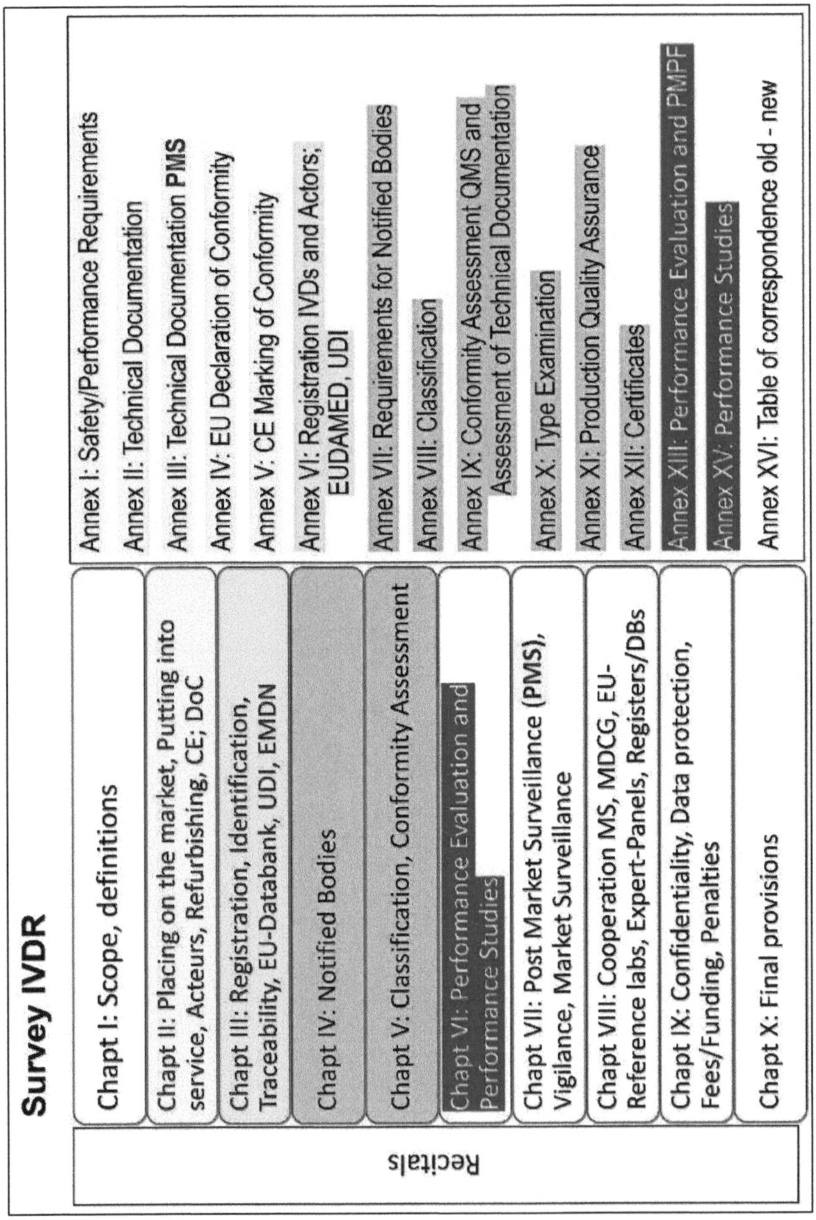

Survey IVDR

Recitals

Chapt I: Scope, definitions	Annex I: Safety/Performance Requirements
Chapt II: Placing on the market, Putting into service, Acteurs, Refurbishing, CE; DoC	Annex II: Technical Documentation
	Annex III: Technical Documentation **PMS**
Chapt III: Registration, Identification, Traceability, EU-Databank, UDI, EMDN	Annex IV: EU Declaration of Conformity
	Annex V: CE Marking of Conformity
Chapt IV: Notified Bodies	Annex VI: Registration IVDs and Actors; EUDAMED, UDI
	Annex VII: Requirements for Notified Bodies
Chapt V: Classification, Conformity Assessment	Annex VIII: Classification
Chapt VI: Performance Evaluation and Performance Studies	Annex IX: Conformity Assessment QMS and Assessment of Technical Documentation
	Annex X: Type Examination
Chapt VII: Post Market Surveillance (PMS), Vigilance, Market Surveillance	Annex XI: Production Quality Assurance
	Annex XII: Certificates
Chapt VIII: Cooperation MS, MDCG, EU-Reference labs, Expert-Panels, Registers/DBs	Annex XIII: Performance Evaluation and PMPF
Chapt IX: Confidentiality, Data protection, Fees/Funding, Penalties	Annex XV: Performance Studies
Chapt X: Final provisions	Annex XVI: Table of correspondence old - new

1.2. The New EU Regulatory System for Medical Devices and IVDs: The Building Principles

(See in particular Fig. 4) Both regulations are based on fundamental legal principles of the EU: the **internal market** concept and **health protection** (which primarily aims at safety and effectiveness, a high level of health protection, a positive clinical benefit/risk ratio according to the state of the art and minimization of risks and side effects).

Both regulations follow basic regulatory principles of the internal market concept[6], as is the

1.2.1. New legal framework for EU product legislation

This is about the new general legal framework for (many) EU product regulations (New Legislative Framework - NLF), which constitute the background philosophy of MDR and IVDR. NLF builds in a modernized form on important legal construction principles, which are essential for the understanding of both regulations: These are the

---

[6] Put forward by Regulation (EC) No 765/2008 and Decision No 768/2008/EC which brought together, in the **New Legislative Framework (NLF)**, all the elements required for a comprehensive regulatory framework to operate effectively for the safety and compliance of industrial products with the requirements adopted to protect the various public interests and for the proper functioning of the single market. On the basis of the *lex specialis* rule, i.e. whenever a matter is regulated by two rules, the more specific one (e.g. the MDR or the IVDR) should be applied first. **Regulation (EC) No 765/2008** established the legal basis for accreditation and market surveillance and consolidated the meaning of the CE marking, thus filling an existing void. **Decision No 768/2008/EC** updated, harmonized and consolidated the various technical instruments already used in existing Union harmonization legislation (not only in New Approach directives): definitions, criteria for the designation and notification of conformity assessment bodies, rules for the designation/notification process, the conformity assessment procedures (modules) and the rules for their use, the safeguard mechanisms, the responsibilities of the economic operators and traceability requirements. The NLF is further explained by the Commission in its **Blue Guide**: 2016/C 272/01 Commission Notice — The 'Blue Guide' on the implementation of EU products rules 2016: https://ec.eu-ropa.eu/growth/content/%E2%80%98blue-guide%E2%80%99-implementation-eu-product-rules-0_en

Fig. 4 MDR-IVDR: Building Principles and Documents - Survey

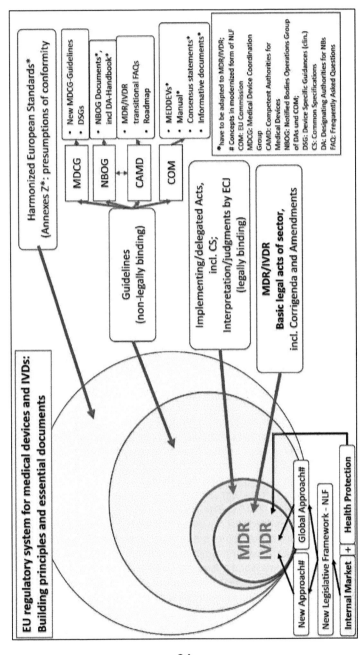

- **New Approach** and the
- **Global Approach**.

1.2.2. The New Approach Under the New Legal Framework

The New Approach is essentially about the following: The two Regulations[7] define in their respective Annexes I checklist-like the **General Safety and Performance Requirements** (GSPR; previously called Essential Requirements - ER) of the MDs or IVDs, which, insofar as they apply to a certain MD/IVD, must be fulfilled by the products on placing on the market or on putting into service. The details to these requirements incl. eventual verification procedures and tests, or on certain processes and procedures of the regulatory system, are provided outside the legal texts by **harmonized European standards**, the references (titles) of which are published in the Official Journal of the EU for the respective Regulation or Directive. These harmonized standards are not binding[8], but contain in their Annexes Z (ZA, ZB, …) very specific **presumptions of conformity** with regard to the GSPR mentioned there for an MD/IVD; i.e. if the manufacturer follows the presumptions of conformity set out in Annexes Z (ZA, ZB,…) of the standards for the fulfilment of certain GSPR, the manufacturer is entitled to a presumption of conformity in this respect from its Notified Body (NB; "European Conformity Assessment Body") or from the market surveillance authority (this presumption may be falsified under certain conditions). The manufacturer may deviate from harmonized standards but must then sufficiently justify his **alternative solutions** for compliance with the relevant GSPR, which usually is associated with increased work load. In the absence of harmonized European standards, current international ISO or IEC standards will often be used alternatively[9]. Harmonized European standards can also provide presumptions of conformity

---

[7] As an example of EU product regulations under the NLF

[8] With the exception of those for harmonized symbols (see EN ISO 15223-1 and related Annexes Z) or on identification colors

[9] At the time of this edition there are only few harmonized standards for MDR and IVDR available; a standardization mandate between the COM and CEN/CENELEC asks to provide a lot of harmonized standards for MDR and IVDR until 27 May 2024. Until that time, global ISO and IEC standards will be an important reference for compliance with GSPR, with a convincing justification. Instead of a reference to GSPR, ISO/IEC standards often contain references to Essential Principles of Safety and Performance in ISO 16142-1:2016 Medical devices —

in important processes and procedures (e.g. quality management systems, clinical investigations, usability, risk management, performance studies).

The Harmonised Standards are drawn up by the European standardization bodies CEN and CENELEC (the latter for the electrotechnical sector) on the basis of standardization mandates of the EU Commission with the help of the standardization bodies of the Member States; they are jointly agreed and harmonized for certain regulations or directives after examination by the Commission. Their references (titles) are published 1-2 times a year in the Official Journal of the EU[10]. European standards are usually developed jointly with the global standards institutions ISO (<> CEN) and IEC (<> CENELEC); however, Appendices Z with the presumptions of conformity are only valid for the Harmonized European Standards.

Further presumptions of conformity can now be provided for certain MD/IVD groups within the framework of both regulations, especially in the clinical area and for Annex XVI products of the MDR, by **Common Specifications, (CS)** in the form of legal acts of the COM.

1.2.3. The Global Approach under the New Legal Framework

The global approach deals with the conformity assessment ("European Pre-market Approval") of products on the basis of modular conformity assessment procedures. These must be selected according to the class of the MD/IVD, derived upon the classification rules of Annex VIII of the MDR/IVDR. For medium and higher classes of the MD/IVD, conformity assessment is carried out by so-called **Notified Bodies (NB)**. Notified Bodies are appointed by the Member States after their proven qualification and competence in a complex, now European supervised procedure for
- **specified product areas,**

Recognized essential principles of safety and performance of medical devices — Part 1: General essential principles and additional specific essential principles for all non-IVD medical devices and guidance on the selection of standards (for MD) or to: ISO 16142-2:2017 Medical devices — Recognized essential principles of safety and performance of medical devices — Part 2: General essential principles and additional specific essential principles for all IVD medical devices and guidance on the selection of standards (for IVD). These ISO principles relate to the Essential principles of GHTF/IMDRF. When trying to relay on Essential principles you have to carefully check differences between the current GSPR of MDR/IVDR against those Essential principles!

[10] Under the reference of the Directive(s) or Regulation(s) concerned

- **specified areas of horizontal technical competence** (e.g. certain technologies (e.g. nanotechnology) or processes (e.g. molecular biological diagnostics), so-called "**horizontal competence codes**"
- **certain conformity assessment modules** (Annexes IX-XI or parts thereof)[11].

The positive completion of approval modules (or certain parts[12] thereof) by the manufacturer is documented by certificates (**NB-certificates**) from the NB (valid for a maximum of 5 years; content of NB-certificates see Annexes XII in both Regulations).

The aim of conformity assessment is the **CE marking of conformity** as a sign of successful EU approval (the correct CE marking is set out in Annex V of both Regulations). The CE marking not only includes proof of compliance with the requirements of MDR/IVDR but also of all EU legal acts that also apply to the product and require CE marking[13] ("inclusive" CE marking).

The CE marking shall be affixed visibly, legibly and indelibly to the device or its sterile packaging. Where such affixing is not possible or not warranted on account of the nature of the device, the CE marking shall be affixed to the packaging. The CE marking shall also appear in any instructions for use and on any sales packaging.

The CE marking is supplemented by the **4-digit identification number** of the NB (if) involved in the conformity assessment[14].

In addition, the manufacturer confirms the conformity of his medical devices/IVDs with the MDR/IVDR and the other EU legal acts applicable to his product, which also require an EU declaration of conformity in addition to the MD/IVDR, by an **EU Declaration of Conformity** ("inclusive" EU Declaration of Conformity) whose basic conditions are described in Art. 19/17 of

---

[11] See chapter 12.4 and 13.4 for selection of suitable NBs; for details see:
COMMISSION IMPLEMENTING REGULATION (EU) 2017/2185 of 23 November 2017 on the list of codes and corresponding types of devices for the purpose of specify-ing the scope of the designation as notified bodies in the field of medical devices under Regulation (EU) 2017/745 of the European Parliament and of the Council and in vitro diagnostic medical devices under Regulation (EU) 2017/746 of the European Parliament and of the Council:
https://eur-lex.europa.eu/legal-content/EN/TXT/?uri=CELEX:32017R2185
[12] E.g. Annex IX is divided into IX.I. QMS and IX.II. Assessment of the Technical Documentation and Annex XI is divided in the MDR into Part A and Part B
[13] See a list of EU legislation in the Blue Guide of the Commission, p.16
[14] See NANDO System of EU COM, see chapters 12.4. and 13.4 in this book

the MDR/IVDR and whose minimum contents are given in Annex IV of both regulations[15].

1.2.4. Plausibility Checks for Successful "European Conformity Assessments" of MD and IVD

These can be based mainly on the following elements:

Tab. 1 Plausibility Check of Successful EU Conformity Assessment for MD and IVD

- **CE marking,**
- **EU Declaration of Conformity,**
- **Identification Number of the Notified Body** (4 digits; if one was involved),
- **Certificate(s) of the Notified Body(s)** (if any) involved**,**
- **Possible control via EUDAMED** (future EU databank)

1.2.5. 'Special Routes' to Market/User

In addition to the main route to CE marking, other **access to the market/user without CE marking** is possible in defined **special routes**, such as (humanitarian) device exemptions or interests of public health (emergency use authorizations, EUA) or patient safety or health by MS or COM[16], in-house production in/for health care facilities in the EU, clinical investigations of MDs or performance studies of IVDs, systems and procedure packs for MD, or as custom made MDs etc. (see chapters 12.2. and 13.2. of this book).

1.3. Market Access Under the New Regulatory Framework: Central Concepts

(making available on the market, placing on the market, putting into service, manufacturer, fully refurbishing)

Art. 5 of both Regulations states [*underscore by author*]:

---

[15] Don't forget the language requirements in the Member States where making available of the product is planned!

[16] Derogation from the conformity assessment procedures: MDR: Art. 59; IVDR: Art. 54

Art. 5 (1): A device may be <u>placed on the market</u> or <u>put into service</u> only if it complies with this Regulation when duly supplied and properly installed, maintained and used in accordance with its intended purpose.

The Blue Guide[17] of the Commission generally states:

"— Union harmonisation legislation applies when the product is placed on the market and to any subsequent operation which constitutes making available until it reaches the end-user."

MDR and IVDR both target the placing on the market and the putting into service. However, it should be noted that the life cycle processes required in MDR and IVDR (e.g. risk management, PMS, vigilance, QMS, clinical evaluation of MD including PMCF, or performance evaluation of IVD including PMPF) cover the entire life cycle, i.e. also the systematic gathering of experience after the initial putting into service of the product (e.g. evaluation of an implant register; long-term studies etc.[18]).

"— Union harmonisation legislation applies to all forms of selling. A product offered in a catalogue or by means of electronic commerce has to comply with Union harmonisation legislation when the catalogue or website directs its offer to the Union market and includes an ordering and shipping system.

—The Union harmonisation legislation applies to newly manufactured products but also to used and second-hand products imported from a third country when they enter the Union market <u>for the first time</u>.

Consider in this context Recital (3) of MDR and IVDR: *This Regulation does not seek to harmonize rules relating to the further making available on the market of medical devices [IVDR: in vitro diagnostic medical devices] after they have already been put into service* (in the EU/EEA - addition by author) *such as in the context of second-hand sales.*

— Union harmonisation legislation applies to finished products[19].

---

[17] See chapter I.2 and https://ec.europa.eu/growth/content/%E2%80%98blue-guide%E2%80%99-implementation-eu-product-rules-0_en

[18] Often referred to as "real world data" as in GHTF/IMDRF or "PLEG" post launch evidence generation as in EUnetHTA.

[19] A variation of this had been introduced under the MDD for e.g. dental crowns or bridges: CE marking of underlying alloys was possible (as deemed appropriate for an industrial manufacturer to demonstrate e.g. biocompatibility and other GSPR), whereas the finished crown or bridge was considered a custom made device without CE-marking (as deemed appropriate for the possibilities of a health handicraft). It will be interesting whether a similar division of requirements would be made possible in the context of the MDR for e.g. 3-D printing of

— A product which has been subject to important changes or overhauls aiming to modify its original performance, purpose or type may be considered as a new product. The person who carries out the changes becomes then the manufacturer with the corresponding obligations."

In this context, you should also pay special attention to Art. 16 of both Regulations (see below!) concerning <u>Relabelers</u> and <u>Repackagers</u>[20] and Art. 23 of the MDR and Art. 20 of the IVDR on <u>parts and components</u> with significant changes.

1.3.1. 'Making Available on the Market'[21] means any supply of a device, other than an investigational device *[IVDR: other than a device for performance study]*, **for distribution, consumption or use on the Union market in the course of a commercial activity, whether in return for payment or free of charge;**

According to the EU Commission's Blue Guide, *"a product is made available on the market when supplied for distribution, consumption or use on the Union market in the course of a commercial activity, whether in return for payment or free of charge. Such supply includes any offer for distribution, consumption or use on the Union market which could result in actual supply (e.g. an invitation to purchase, advertising campaigns).*

— <u>The concept of making available refers to each individual product.</u>[22]

The central role that the concept of making available plays in Union harmonisation legislation is related to the fact that all economic operators in the supply-chain have traceability obligations and need to have an active role in ensuring that only compliant products circulate on the Union market. The

---

implants, with a division into industrial producers of 3-D printers, related software and related printing materials (with CE-marking demonstrating conformity with GSPR, including safety and effectiveness for specific health care applications) versus in house producers in health care as custom made manufacturers. See here also: MDCG 2021-3: Questions and Answers on Custom-Made Devices: https://ec.europa.eu/health/medical-devices-sector/new-regulations/guidance-mdcg-endorsed-documents-and-other-guidance_en

[20] See also: MDCG 2021-26: Q&A on repackaging & relabelling activities under Article 16 of Regulation (EU) 2017/745 and Regulation (EU) 2017/746: https://ec.europa.eu/health/medical-devices-sector/new-regulations/guidance-mdcg-endorsed-documents-and-other-guidance_en

[21] MDR: Art. 2 (27); IVDR: Art. 2 Nr. 20

[22] Underlined by author

concept of making available refers to each individual product, not to a type of product, and whether it was manufactured as an individual unit or in series. - The making available of a product supposes an offer or an agreement (written or verbal) between two or more legal or natural persons for the transfer of ownership, possession or any other right concerning the product in question after the stage of manufacture has taken place. The transfer does not necessarily require the physical handover of the product. This transfer can be for payment or free of charge, and it can be based on any type of legal instrument. Thus, a transfer of a product is considered to have taken place, for instance, in the circumstances of sale, loan, hire, leasing and gift. Transfer of ownership implies that the product is intended to be placed at the disposal of another legal or natural person."

......

1.3.2. 'Placing on the Market'[23] means <u>the first making available of a device</u>, other than an investigational device *[IVDR: other than a device for performance study]*, **on the Union market;**

The Blue Guide explains further:

"— Products made available on the market must comply with the applicable Union harmonisation legislation at the moment of placing on the market. This calls for a simultaneous application of various legislative acts which apply to a given product. Accordingly, the product has to be designed and manufactured in accordance with all applicable Union harmonisation legislation, as well as to undergo the conformity assessment procedures according to all applicable legislation, unless otherwise provided for[24].
- The operation is reserved either for a manufacturer or an importer, i.e. the manufacturer and the importer are the only economic operators who place products on the market. When a manufacturer or an importer supplies a product to a distributor or an end-user for the first time, the operation is al-

---

[23] MDR: Art. 2 (28); IVDR: Art. 2 no. 21; underlining by author
[24] See also chapters 12.1 and 13.1 in this book on prior clarification of the whole legislative portfolio a product has to match

ways labelled in legal terms as 'placing on the market'. Any subsequent operation, for instance, from a distributor to distributor or from a distributor to an end-user is defined as making available.

- As for 'making available', the <u>concept of placing on the market refers to each individual product</u>[25], not to a type of product, and whether it was manufactured as an individual unit or in series.

- Placing a product on the market requires an offer or an agreement (written or verbal) between two or more legal or natural persons for the transfer of ownership, possession or any other property right concerning the product in question after the stage of manufacture has taken place. This transfer could be for payment or free of charge. It does not require the physical handover of the product.

- The placing on the market is the most decisive point in time concerning the application of the Union harmonised legislation. When made available on the market, products must be in compliance with the Union harmonisation legislation applicable at the time of placing on the market. Accordingly, new products manufactured in the Union and all products imported from third countries — whether new or used — must meet the provisions of the applicable Union harmonisation legislation when placed on the market, i.e. when made available for the first time on the Union market.

- The making available or putting into service can only take place when the product complies with the provisions of all applicable Union harmonisation legislation at the time of its placing on the market.

- Products offered for sale by online operators based in the EU are considered to have been placed on the Union market, regardless of who placed them on the market (the online operator, the importer, etc.). Products offered for sale online by sellers based outside the EU are considered to be placed on the Union market if sales are specifically targeted at EU consumers or other end-users."

- see more details concerning online operators in the Blue Guide (p.21ff);
Important: MDR and IVDR in their Articles 6 directly refer to "Distance sales".

---

[25] Underlined by author

- Finally, the Blue Guide demonstrates examples when placing on the market is not considered to take place (p.21).

For more information on "Placing on the market" in case of disputed questions of "whether" and "when" please refer to the Informative Document (Guidance) of the EU Commission: PLACING ON THE MARKET OF MEDICAL DEVICES[26].

> **1.3.3. 'Putting into Service' means the stage at which a device, other than an investigational device** *[IVDR: other than a device for performance study]*, **has been made available to the final user as being ready for use on the Union market for the first time for its intended purpose[27];**

"- Putting into service takes place at the moment of first use within the Union by the end user for the purposes for which it was intended. This concept is also applied for MDs and IVDs.

- Where the product is put into service by an employer for use by his employees, the employer is considered as the end-user."

Important: Art. 5 (1 and 4) of both Regulations:

1. A device may be placed on the market or <u>put into service</u> only if it complies with this Regulation when duly supplied and properly installed, maintained and used in accordance with its intended purpose.

....

4.<u>Devices that are manufactured and used within health institutions shall be considered as having been put into service.</u>

With regard to **in-house production** in/for health institutions in the EU see specifically Art. 5 (5) of both Regulations![28]

> **1.3.4. 'Manufacturer' means a natural or legal person who manufactures or fully refurbishes a device or has a device designed, manufactured or fully refurbished, and markets that device under its name or trademark[29];**

---

[26] This interpretative document has been elaborated in line with the NLF, but under the MD-Directives. http://ec.europa.eu/DocsRoom/documents/10265/attachments/1/translations
[27] MDR: Art. 2 (29); IVDR: Art. 2 no 22
[28] See also a prolongation of certain transition periods for this IVD-in-house production by regulation (EU) 2022/112
[29] MDR: Art. 2 (30); IVDR: Art. 2 no 23

In both Regulations the obligations of the manufacturer are now explicitly listed in Art. 10. Furthermore Art. 16 of both Regulations state:

1. A distributor, importer or other natural or legal person shall assume the obligations incumbent on manufacturers if it does any of the following:

(a) makes available on the market a device under its name, registered trade name or registered trade mark, except in cases where a distributor or importer enters into an agreement with a manufacturer whereby the manufacturer is identified as such on the label and is responsible for meeting the requirements placed on manufacturers in this Regulation (author: means MDR or IVDR)*;*

(b) changes the intended purpose of a device already placed on the market or put into service;

(c) modifies a device already placed on the market or put into service in such a way that compliance with the applicable requirements may be affected.

...

Relabellers and Repackagers: see section 1.3.7.

...

1.3.5. 'Fully Refurbishing' for the purposes of the definition of manufacturer, means the complete rebuilding of a device already placed on the market or put into service, or the making of a new device from used devices, to bring it into conformity with this Regulation, combined with the assignment of a new lifetime to the refurbished device[30];

Please also have a look in this context on Art. 17 of MDR concerning single use devices and their reprocessing and the corresponding national legislations and on: Commission Implementing Regulation (EU) 2020/1207 of 19 August 2020 laying down rules for the application of Regulation (EU) 2017/745 of the European Parliament and of the Council as regards **common specifications for the reprocessing of single-use devices,** as well as on national legislation.

---

[30] MDR: Art. 2 (31); IVDR: Art. 2 no 24

1.3.6. Distance Sales

MDR/IVDR: Art. 6 (1): *A device offered by means of information society services[31], to a natural or legal person established in the Union shall comply with this Regulation.*

2. Without prejudice to national law regarding the exercise of the medical profession, a device that is not placed on the market but used in the context of a commercial activity, whether in return for payment or free of charge, for the provision of a diagnostic or therapeutic service offered by means of information society services[32] or by other means of communication, directly or through intermediaries, to a natural or legal person established in the Union shall comply with this Regulation.

3. Upon request by a competent authority, any natural or legal person offering a device in accordance with paragraph 1 or providing a service in accordance with paragraph 2 shall make available a copy of the EU declaration of conformity of the device concerned.

4. A Member State may, on grounds of protection of public health, require a provider of information society services[33], to cease its activity.

On the activities of online providers, see also the Blue Guide.

1.3.7. Relabellers and Repackagers

Important considerations for **Relabellers and Repackagers**: (we are still on Art. 16 of both Regulations):

Art. 16.1.: see section 1.3.4. above

Art. 16.2. For the purposes of point (c) of paragraph 1, the following shall not be considered to be a modification of a device that could affect its compliance with the applicable requirements:

---

[31] as defined in point (b) of Article 1(1) of Directive (EU) 2015/1535: DIRECTIVE (EU) 2015/1535 OF THE EUROPEAN PARLIAMENT AND OF THE COUNCIL of 9 September 2015 laying down a procedure for the provision of information in the field of technical regulations and of rules on Information Society services (codification); https://eur-lex.europa.eu/legal-content/EN/TXT/PDF/?uri=CELEX:32015L1535&from=en

[32] as footnote above

[33] As footnotes above

(a) provision, including translation, of the information supplied by the manufacturer, in accordance with Section 23 of Annex I [IVDR: Section 20 of Annex I], relating to a device already placed on the market and of further information which is necessary in order to market the device in the relevant Member State;

(b) changes to the outer packaging of a device already placed on the market, including a change of pack size, if the repackaging is necessary in order to market the device in the relevant Member State and if it is carried out in such conditions that the original condition of the device cannot be affected by it. In the case of devices placed on the market in sterile condition, it shall be presumed that the original condition of the device is adversely affected if the packaging that is necessary for maintaining the sterile condition is opened, damaged or otherwise negatively affected by the repackaging.

3. A distributor or importer that carries out any of the activities mentioned in points (a) and (b) of paragraph 2 shall indicate on the device or, where that is impracticable, on its packaging or in a document accompanying the device, the activity carried out together with its name, registered trade name or registered trade mark, registered place of business and the address at which it can be contacted, so that its location can be established. Distributors and importers shall ensure that they have in place a quality management system that includes procedures which ensure that the translation of information is accurate and up-to-date, and that the activities mentioned in points (a) and (b) of paragraph 2 are performed by a means and under conditions that preserve the original condition of the device and that the packaging of the repackaged device is not defective, of poor quality or untidy. The quality management system shall cover, inter alia, procedures ensuring that the distributor or importer is informed of any corrective action taken by the manufacturer in relation to the device in question in order to respond to safety issues or to bring it into conformity with this Regulation.

4. At least 28 days prior to making the relabelled or repackaged device available on the market, distributors or importers carrying out any of the activities mentioned in points (a) and (b) of paragraph 2 shall inform the manufacturer and the competent authority of the Member State in which they plan to make the device available of the intention to make the relabelled or repackaged device available and, upon request, shall provide the manufacturer and the competent authority with a sample or mock-up of the relabelled or repackaged device, including any translated label and instructions for use. Within the same period of 28 days, the distributor or importer shall submit to the competent authority a certificate, issued by a notified body designated for the type of devices that are subject to activities mentioned in points (a) and (b) of paragraph 2, attesting that the quality management system of the distributer or importer complies with the requirements laid down in paragraph 3.

See also: See also: MDCG 2021-26: Q&A on repackaging & relabelling activities under Article 16 of Regulation (EU) 2017/745 and Regulation (EU) 2017/746: https://ec.europa.eu/health/medical-devices-sector/new-regulations/guidance-mdcg-endorsed-documents-and-other-guidance_en

1.4. Important Documents of the Regulatory System

(see Fig. 4)

1.4.1. The Main Legal Acts for MD and IVD

- **Regulation (EU) 2017/745 concerning medical devices (MDR), and**
- **Regulation (EU) 2017/746 on in vitro diagnostic medical devices (IVDR)**

Please consider here any Corrigenda and Amendments to these Regulations[34]:

- Corrigendum of 5 May 2019 to Regulation (EU) 2017/745 on medical devices, amending Directive 2001/83/EC, Regulation (EC) No 178/2002 and Regulation (EC) No 1223/2009 and repealing Directives 90/385/EEC and 93/42/EEC.
  This 1st Corr. of MDR brings smaller corrections for clinical investigations, clarifications and adaptations for sampling procedures of the technical documentation in the Annexes VII and IX in the course of conformity assessment, together with a clarification for the classification of accessories in Annex VIII.
- Corrigendum of 27 December 2019 to Regulation (EU) 2017/745 on medical devices, amending Directive 2001/83/EC, Regulation (EC) No 178/2002 and Regulation (EC) No 1223/2009 and repealing Directives

---

[34] See here: https://ec.europa.eu/health/medical-devices-sector/new-regulations_en

90/385/EEC and 93/42/EEC.
This 2nd Corrigendum of MDR contains important changes to transition periods for certain Class I MDs under the MDR, see chapt. I.6. in this book for details. There are also further clarifications to the registration obligations and
corrections to some false references.

- Corrigendum of 5 May 2019 to Regulation (EU) 2017/746 on in vitro diagnostic medical devices, repealing Directive 98/79/EC and Commission decision
  2010/227/EU
  This 1st Corrigendum to the IVDR contains corrections to misleading provisions
  for performance studies, adaptations with regard to sampling procedures for
  the technical documentation during conformity assessment in Annexes VII
  and IX.
- Corrigendum of 27 December 2019 to Regulation (EU) 2017/746 on
  in vitro diagnostic medical devices, repealing Directive 98/79/EC and
  Commission decision 2010/227/EU.
  This 2nd Corrigendum gives corrections of some redactional errors, clarifications to registration obligations in the transition from IVD-Directive to IVDR
  and a clarification concerning classification acc. to Annex VIII for diagnosis of
  feto-maternal blood group incompatibilities.

- REGULATION (EU) 2020/561 OF THE EUROPEAN PARLIAMENT AND OF THE
  COUNCIL of 23 April 2020 amending Regulation (EU) 2017/745 on medical devices as regards the date of application of some of its provisions.
  **This amending regulation postponed the date of application of the MDR by 1
  year to 26 May 2021**; it also stipulates that for certain Class I (excluding Im
  and Is) medical devices of Directive 93/42/EEC, for which referral to a Notified
  Body is now necessary under the MDR and for which an EU Declaration of
  Conformity was issued before 26.5.2021 under Directive 93/42/EEC and further conditions are fulfilled (see chapter 1.6. in this book), these may be
  placed on the market or put into or put into service until 26.5.2024. Furthermore, Art. 59 is amended in such a way that (emergency use) Exemptions
  from the Member States and the COM - in view of the COVID crisis - can already be extended under the MD Directive 93/42/EEC to the Union. Amendments from the 2nd Corr. of MDR are confirmed or clarified.
- Regulation (EU) 2022/112 of the European Parliament and of the Council of 25 January 2022 amending Regulation (EU) 2017/746 as regards

transitional provisions for certain in vitro diagnostic medical devices and the deferred application of conditions for in-house devices[35]

1.4.2. Implementing and Delegated Acts of the COM

Besides the two basic regulations and their Corrigenda and Amendments, we can expect a wealth of implementing legislation from COM, either as **implementing acts or delegated acts** based on authorisation in the regulations. This includes the future **Common Specifications (CS)** with specific requirements, especially for clinical aspects (clinical investigations, clinical evaluation, PMCF of specific types of MD; performance studies, performance evaluations and PMPF of specific types of IVD) of certain high-risk product types, but also of Annex XVI products.

Already issued as CS:

- Commission Implementing Regulation (EU) 2020/1207 of 19 August 2020 laying down rules for the application of Regulation (EU) 2017/745 of the European Parliament and of the Council as regards **common specifications for the reprocessing of single-use devices**

- Commission Implementing Regulation (EU) 2021/2226 of 14 December 2021 laying down rules for the application of Regulation (EU) 2017/745 of the European Parliament and of the Council as regards **electronic instructions for use of medical devices**

- Commission Implementing Regulation (EU) 2021/2078 of 26 November 2021 laying down rules for the application of Regulation (EU) 2017/745 of the European Parliament and of the Council as regards the **European Database on Medical Devices (Eudamed)**

- Commission Implementing Regulation (EU) 2020/1207 of 19 August 2020 laying down rules for the application of Regulation (EU) 2017/745 of the European Parliament and of the Council as regards **common specifications for the reprocessing of single-use devices**

- Commission Implementing Regulation (EU) 2017/2185 of 23 November 2017 on the **codes for the designation of notified bodies** in medical devices under Regulation (EU) 2017/745 and in vitro diagnostic medical devices under Regulation (EU)

---

[35] https://eur-lex.europa.eu/legal-content/EN/TXT/?uri=uris-erv:OJ.L_.2022.019.01.0003.01.ENG

2017/746;

(This will be important for the search of suitable NBs, see Annex I with the codes for MDR and Annex II with the codes for IVDR; see chapters XII.4 and XIII.4 in this book)

- Commission Implementing Decision (EU) 2019/1396 of 10 September 2019 laying down the rules for the application of Regulation (EU) 2017/745 of the European Parliament and of the Council as regards the **designation of expert panels in the field of medical devices**

- Commission Implementing Decision (EU) 2019/939 of 6 June 2019 **designating issuing entities designated to operate a system for the assignment of Unique Device Identifiers (UDIs)** in the field of medical devices

(In the annex, the EU Commission has officially designated the following UDI issuing entities for an initial period of five years: (a) GS1 AISBL (b) Health
Industry Business Communications Council (HIBCC) (c) ICCBBA (d) Information Centre for proprietary medicinal products - IFA GmbH.)

- COMMISSION IMPLEMENTING DECISION (EU) 2020/437 of 24 March 2020 concerning harmonised standards for medical devices in support of Council Directive 93/42/EEC;

- COMMISSION IMPLEMENTING DECISION (EU) 2019/1396 of 10 September 2019 laying down detailed rules for the implementation of Regulation (EU) 2017/745 of the European Parliament and of the Council as regards the **designation of expert panels for medical devices**.

- COMMISSION IMPLEMENTING DECISION (EU) 2021/1182

of 16 July 2021 on the **harmonised standards for medical devices** drafted in support of Regulation (EU) 2017/745 of the European Parliament and of the Council[36]

COMMISSION IMPLEMENTING DECISION (EU) 2021/1195 of 19 July 2021

on the **harmonised standards for in vitro diagnostic medical devices** drafted in support of Regulation (EU) 2017/746 of the European Parliament and of the Council[37]

---

[36] See current publications and a summary list of HN for MDR: https://ec.europa.eu/growth/single-market/european-standards/harmonised-standards/medical-devices_en

[37] See current publications and a summary list of HN for IVDR: https://ec.europa.eu/growth/single-market/european-standards/harmonised-standards/iv-diagnostic-medical-devices_en

Please also note that the following implementing legislation of the COM for the Medical Devices Directive is, until further notice, to be considered implementing legislation under the MDR:
- COMMISSION REGULATION (EU) No. 722/2012 of 8 August 2012
2012 concerning particular requirements as regards the requirements laid down in Council Directives 90/385/EEC and 93/42/EEC with respect to active implantable medical devices and medical devices **manufactured utilising tissues of animal origin**.
[Protection against TSEs (transmissible spongiform encephalopathies, like BSE, scrapie, CJD and vCJD]
Further implementation legislation will follow; the prioritization can be anticipated on the basis of the the rolling plan of the COM[38] and the roadmap on the CAMD homepage[39]; within the framework of regulatory compliance, these must be tracked under the QMS as well as any **Amendments and Corrigenda of the underlying MDR and IVDR**.

1.4.3 Monopoly of legal interpretation of EU law

The (legally binding) monopoly on interpretation of EU law is the responsibility of the European Court of Justice and **Judgements and Decisions of the ECJ[40]** must also be carefully pursued.

1.4.4. Non-legally binding Guidance

Due to the strong heterogeneity of the product area, a dense, non-legally binding set of guidelines (guidance) is being and has been developed for the medical device/IVD sector.

---

[38] See https://ec.europa.eu/health/document/download/6d1552b6-b52a-484c-80dc-3616959cedf1_en
[39] See https://www.camd-europe.eu/
[40] See: https://curia.europa.eu/jcms/jcms/j_6/en/ ; (search form) http://curia.europa.eu/juris/recherche.jsf?pro=&nat=or&oqp=&dates=&lg=&language=en&jur=C%2CT%2CF&cit=none%252CC%252CCJ%252CR%252C2008E%252C%252C%252C%252C%252C%252C%252C%252C%252Ctrue%252Cfalse%252Cfalse&td=%3BALL&pcs=Oor&avg=&mat=or&jge=&for=&cid=707816

MDCG (Medical Device Coordination Group) is now the originator of most of the guidance (MDCG-documents) for the new Regulations[41]; there may also be still guidance from the COM or the CAMD.

1.4.4.1. MDCG guidance[42]

currently centres on these issues for the MDR/IVDR:

Clinical investigation and evaluation; Covid-19; custom made devices; EU-DAMED; European Medical Device Nomenclature (EMDN); New technologies (incl. software); IVDs; Notified bodies; UDI; other topics.

Ongoing MDCG guidance is indicated here: https://ec.europa.eu/health/document/download/b14e2630-6d0a-4f02-a494-d0a89c48e7a4_en

Important to notice: MDR/IVDR request the NBs to consider guidance and best practice documents adopted in the framework of these Regulations during conformity assessment[43]. This should also be a strong incentive for manufacturers to stick to these documents wherever possible.

1.4.4.2. Guidance documents of the COM

Under the Directives, the COM had developed a lot of guidance documents, jointly agreed by all stakeholders, organised in various EU working groups, and approved under the patronage of the Medical Device Expert Group (MDEG). These guidances will have to be adjusted to the MDR/IVDR, then probably as MDCG-documents.

COM guidance is available at the COM homepage in different formats[44]:

The **MEDDEVs** (Medical Device Guidelines), e.g. on demarcation issues (pharmaceuticals) for MD and IVD, clinical evaluation, vigilance still have considerable value under MDR/IVDR, but check carefully against the text of the regulations!

The **Manual**[45]: with joint stakeholder "decisions" on individual cases of qualification (delineation) and classification of MD and IVD under the Directives; please consider the many changes to the classification of MDs and esp. IVDs

---

[41] https://ec.europa.eu/health/md_sector/new_regulations/guidance_en

[42] https://ec.europa.eu/health/md_sector/new_regulations/guidance_en

[43] See Annex VII of both regulations

[44] https://ec.europa.eu/health/md_sector/current_directives_en

[45] https://ec.europa.eu/health/sites/health/files/md_topics-interest/docs/md_borderline_manual_05_2019_en.pdf

under the new Regulations, rather look at the new MDCG-guidance for classification of MDs and IVDs; current entries of the manual will probably stay as they are under the Directives, except those for classification of IVDs, which is completely outdated; only new entries may automatically target the MDR/IVDR purposes.

Interpretative documents[46] (e.g. Placing on the market; own brand labellers) and **consensus statements** (e.g. Class I medical devices; custom made devices; IVD rare blood groups).

1.4.4.3. Guidance by Member States-Working Groups:

NBOG[47] **best practice guides, NBOG checklists, NBOG forms**: Guidance documents from the Designating Authorities of MS on best practice for NB and the implementation of conformity assessment procedures. In addition to those for the previous Directives, including the **Designating Authorities Handbook**, a whole series of documents have already been developed for the designation of the NBs under the new Regulations (as MDCG documents or as NBOG Best Practice Guides[48])

This whole network of (non-legally binding) guidance documents will be revised in the coming years for the purposes of the new EU regulations. The rolling plan of the MDCG[49]/COM and the CAMD roadmap are the best way to determine the target direction and current priorities. The patronage of many guidelines will pass to the MDCG (Medical Devices Coordination Group)[50].

These developments, which are also very important for the manufacturer, should be actively and systematically anticipated and monitored under his QMS for regulatory compliance purposes (change management!).

---

[46] https://ec.europa.eu/health/md_sector/current_directives_en

[47] NBOG: Notified Body Operations Group; https://www.nbog.eu/

[48] See also: https://ec.europa.eu/health/document/download/b14e2630-6d0a-4f02-a494-d0a89c48e7a4_en and: https://ec.europa.eu/health/md_sector/new_regulations/guidance_en

[49] https://ec.europa.eu/health/document/download/b14e2630-6d0a-4f02-a494-d0a89c48e7a4_en

[50] http://ec.europa.eu/growth/sectors/medical-devices/guidance_en

See also Fig. 4 EU regulatory system for MDs and IVDs: key documents and construction principles

1.4.4.4. Guidance documents of GHTF/IMDRF[51]:

These global, non-legally binding guidance documents may be useful for global ambitions of manufacturers. There is a commitment of the COM to adjust the EU-system in future to some of these global guidelines, as already has been seen in the preparation of MDR/IVDR. Current areas of specific interest may be IMDRF guidelines on PMS, Real World Data (e.g. implant register evaluations), the Medical Device Single Audit Program (MDSAP) or the Codes für vigilance reports [www.imdrf.org]. Always have a careful look at EU legislation and MDCG guidance first!

1.4.5. Harmonised European Standards

In addition to the Common Specifications (which are implementing legislation of the COM), the Harmonized European Standards (HN for harmonised

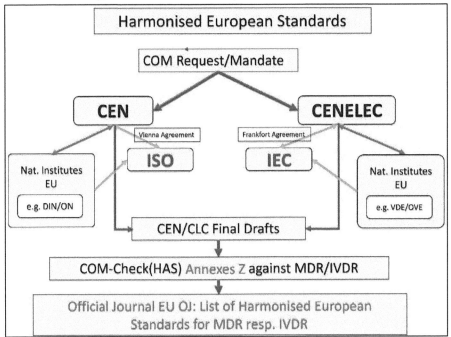

Fig. 5 Harmonised European Standards

---

51 https://www.imdrf.org/

norms; see Fig. 5) in their Annexes Z also grant **presumptions of conformity** for certain requirements of the Regulations (and previously the Directives), in particular also the requirements of Annex I (General Safety and Performance Requirements - GSPR).

The lists of Harmonised European Standards (titles only!) for the new Regulations, as well as for the previous Directives, are published 1-2 times a year in the **Official Journal of the EU**, after review by COM[52]. Note: Standards may also be de-harmonized with new findings.

The previous harmonised standards must now also be adapted to the new Regulations and harmonised under these again[53]! Please monitor these developments closely as a manufacturer under your QMS and also take these into account in the context of your change management[54]. The harmonised standards are available in their respective language versions from the national standards bodies (usually you will be charged).

---

[52] See summary list of HN as pdf for MDR: https://ec.europa.eu/docsroom/documents/48579 ; see summary list of HN for IVDR: https://ec.europa.eu/docsroom/documents/48577

[53] At the time of this edition short lists of harmonized standards for MDR and IVDR have been published, and work will go on; a standardization mandate between the COM and CEN/CENELEC has been issued, to provide a lot of harmonized standards for MDR and IVDR until 27 May 2024. Until that time, global ISO and IEC standards will be an important possible reference for compliance with GSPR, after a careful check against the provisions of MDR/IVDR. Instead of a reference to GSPR, ISO/IEC standards often contain references to Essential Principles of Safety and Performance as given in: (for MDs) ISO 16142-1:2016 Medical devices — Recognized essential principles of safety and performance of medical devices — Part 1: General essential principles and additional specific essential principles for all non-IVD medical devices and guidance on the selection of standards or to: (for IVDs) ISO 16142-2:2017 Medical devices — Recognized essential principles of safety and performance of medical devices — Part 2: General essential principles and additional specific essential principles for all IVD medical devices and guidance on the selection of standards. These ISO principles relate to the Essential principles of GHTF/IMDRF (which had been largely copied from the European Essential Requirements under the Directives). When trying to relay on Essential principles you have to carefully check differences between the current GSPR of MDR/IVDR against those Essential principles!

[54] E.g. in case a manufacturer loses previously used presumptions of conformity for his product(s) with new versions of a harmonized standard

Examples of important (harmonised or not yet harmonised**) European standards for the medical device directives** (to be adapted to Regulations!)**:** Please note in the most recent publication in the Official Journal of the EU the current versions (dates) of the standards and the end of the transition period of the outdated previous version; this has to be followed by the manufacturer under the QMS [regulatory compliance with regard to use of presumptions of conformity in change management):

EN ISO 10993 series: Biological evaluation of medical devices (particularly important as a starter: Part 1: Evaluation and testing within the framework of a risk management procedure) [for the selection of necessary tests for biocompatibility and their algorithms].

EN ISO 11135-1: Sterilization of healthcare products - Ethylene oxide - Part 1: Requirements for the development, validation and control of the application of a sterilization process for medical devices

EN ISO 11137 series: Sterilization of health care products - Radiation

EN ISO 11607 series: Packaging for medical devices to be sterilized in the final packaging

EN ISO 13408 series: Aseptic manufacture of healthcare products

EN ISO 13485 Medical devices - Quality management systems - Requirements for regulatory purposes

EN ISO 14155 Clinical investigation of medical devices for human subjects - Good clinical practice

EN ISO 14630 Non-active surgical implants - General requirements

EN ISO 14937 Sterilization of health care products -
General requirements for the characterization of a sterilizing agent and for the development, validation and control of the application of a sterilization process for medical devices

EN ISO 14971 Medical devices - Application of risk management
on medical devices

EN ISO 15223-1 Medical devices - Symbols to be used with medical device labels, labelling and information to be supplied - Part 1: General requirements

EN ISO 15883 series: washer-disinfectors

EN ISO 17664 series: Sterilization of medical devices - Information to be provided by the manufacturer

EN ISO 17665 series: Sterilization of health care products -
Moist heat (steam sterilization!)

EN ISO TR 20416 Medical devices — Post-market surveillance for manufacturers

EN ISO 20417 Medical devices — Information to be supplied by the manufacturer

EN 60601 Parts 1-Series: Medical electrical equipment -[currently 1-11]

General safety requirements including essential performance characteristics

EN 60601 Parts 2 Series: Medical Electrical Equipment -

Special requirements for safety, including the

essential performance features of .... (special species/groups of MD [currently > 80, drafts already reach up to more than 80!]

EN 62304 Medical Device Software - Software Life Cycle Processes

EN 62366 Medical devices - Application of suitability for use to medical devices; ('usability')

1.4.6. Anticipation and Monitoring of Later Changes to Legal and In-terpretational Documents

In the pursue of **change management** under the manufacturer's QMS, it is crucial to keep a watchful eye on forthcoming changes to the legal basis and relevant legally binding and non-binding interpretations and to new (versions of) harmonized standards (HN) and to anticipate, monitor and react in a timely manner:

Most important are

- possible changes to the basic legal acts MDR and IVDR, which may take the form of **corrections[55] or amendments[56]**. These will be published in the Official Journal (OJ) of the EU and will be referenced (and usually drafts will earlier be announced) at the COM's homepage of the sector. Drafts of amendments may be seen earlier in official consultation procedures to the public and stakeholders.

- **Implementing and delegated Acts** to MDR/IVDR may be issued by the COM following the legal provisions in MDR/IVDR. The next planned steps are currently announced in the **rolling plan** of the COM[57] and the **roadmap** of the Competent Authorities for Medical

---

[55] Sometimes only for some language versions

[56] See currently Regulation (EU) 2021/561 for MDR and Regulation (EU) 2022/112 for IVDR; see also: https://ec.europa.eu/health/medical-devices-sector/new-regulations_en

[57] https://ec.europa.eu/docsroom/documents/31902

Devices (CAMD)[58]. Please note that the **Common Specifications (CS)** will also belong to these Acts and will deliver presumptions of conformity for MDR/IVDR (mainly in the clinical area for MDs, the performance area for IVDs and will be mandatory for Annex XVI MDs).

- Legally binding **Judgments and Opinions of the Court of Justice of the European Union** ("ECJ") within its monopoly of interpretation and its role as the supreme guardian of European Union legality[59].

Direct search, setting automatic alarms and getting hints through frequent networking with stakeholder organisations and competent authorities and subscribing for relevant newsletters will help to be always on the ball.

With regard to **non-legally binding interpretation** through guidelines, you should primarily look at new guidelines by the MDCG (see rolling plan of MDCG[60]), (forthcoming or revised) guidelines of the COM, and of the Competent Authorities of the Member States (CAMD[61]). All existing 'old' guidances have now to be adapted to MDR/IVDR. Global strategic developments can be seen in GHTF/IMDRF-guidance documents:

Insights for anticipation of developments at legal or guidance level can be gathered via contacts with national competent authorities' networks (e.g. "Jour fixes", national mirror groups and newsletters) or stakeholder networks, or the COM, see Link list. The drafts of new guidance documents are generated and further processed in the relevant working groups (now under the MDCG) and may be influenced via stakeholder organisations (industry, health care institutions and professionals, health insurances, patient organisations) participating there. The near future work program of MDCG can be seen at the **rolling plan of the MDCG[62]** and the **COM** and the **CAMD roadmap**.

---

[58] https://www.camd-europe.eu/
[59] https://curia.europa.eu/jcms/jcms/j_6/en/
[60] https://ec.europa.eu/health/document/download/b14e2630-6d0a-4f02-a494-d0a89c48e7a4_en
[61] https://www.camd-europe.eu/
[62] *Present guidelines under:* https://ec.europa.eu/health/medical-devices-sector/new-regulations/guidance-mdcg-endorsed-documents-and-other-guidance_en *; planned MDCG*

If you are interested in the global strategic regulatory developments, it might be useful to screen guideline development at IMDRF. These guidelines are all accessible via the IMDRF homepage (also the "old" GHTF guidance). The drafts of forthcoming guidance are presented for global consultation via the various regions, so you might influence them via your region.

1.5. Regulatory Compliance – A Short Walkthrough Along the Product Life Cycle

(see Fig. 6 for MDR and Fig. 7 for IVDR; for both: Tab. 2)
Fig. 6 and 7 show you how the important steps and processes of the regulatory product life-cycle are aligned within the obligatory QMS of the manufacturer. Hope you'll never get lost within the new regulatory system!

QMS and process build-up :
Ideally any product development would start under the QMS of the manufacturer and, as a future MD or IVD, would be piloted along the life-cycle by validated processes under the QMS, including the most important life-cycle processes, like risk management system (RMS), technical, preclinical and clinical evaluation (for MDs) and technical, analytical and clinical performance evaluation (for IVDs), post market surveillance system (PMS), Vigilance.

Most important (life-cycle) processes would start with their respective plans. These plans would indicate the goals, objectives, ressources, controls and necessary documentation of the whole process within the regulatory system. It would also indicate the validated methods to reach those goals and objectives, e.g. the sources, methods and ressources to generate, collect, appraise, analyse and document necessary data and how to draw the important conclusions from this active and systematic exercise. Conclusions could be indications for improvements, changes to the process a/o product a/o intended purpose, CAPAs or even FSCA a/o changes to documentation (e.g. TD, risk management documentation, clinical evaluation report, performance evaluation report etc). Usually a formal instructive report on the exercise has to be issued, indicating whether the goals have been reached, any gaps still

---

documents under: https://ec.europa.eu/health/document/download/b14e2630-6d0a-4f02-a494-d0a89c48e7a4_en

open and any further action needed. As most processes are life cycle processes, the activities under the process have to be continued over the life cycle, such as under the PMCF or PMPF or risk management to update the conclusions and reports. These updated reports will be subject to control mechanisms, like management reviews, audits by NBs or inspections by Competent Authorities or may even go public. You may see these processes as following the classical PDCA-cycle (Plan-Do-Check-Act).

While this is a "routine" matter of course for established manufacturers who already manage a product portfolio, MD/IVD research projects, start-ups and spin-offs may have to establish their processes "on the run" and accomplish their system build-up with the QMS stepwise. This clear build-up of all necessary processes will pay substantially for all further enlargement of the product portfolio!

Fig. 6 Regulatory pathway MDR

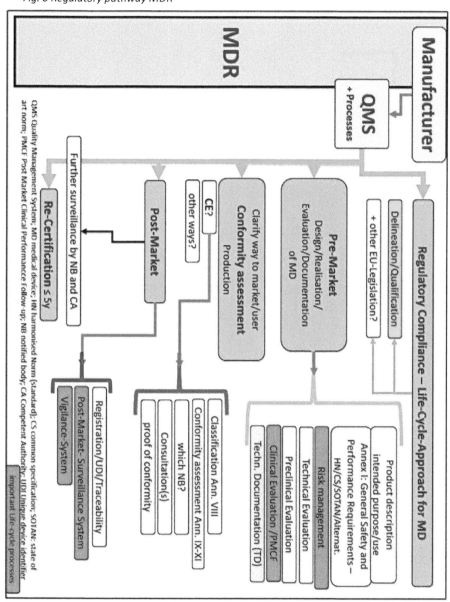

Fig. 7 Regulatory pathway IVDR

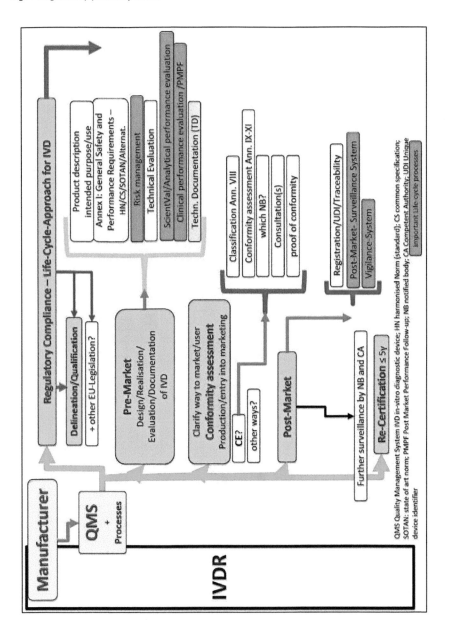

Premarket regulatory milestones:

Important milestones will be the **qualification** exercise (assurance, that the product falls under the MDR or IVDR[63]). If this is confirmed, an investigation, if other Community (or national) legislation applies, esp. those which require CE-marking a/o the obligation to issue an EU Declaration of Conformity. This is important to have on screen from the beginning the **full regulatory spectrum to fulfil**.

Technical development will have to be accompanied and piloted by the processes (incl. **Risk Management**, under the specific RM-plan for this device) to fulfil the **General Safety and Performance Requirements (GSPR) of Annex I** applicable to the device (see chapter V of this book).

After **technical evaluation, preclinical evaluation** of MDs (see chapter V.3 and Annex I.II.10-13) and **analytical performance evaluation** of IVD [as part of the overall performance evaluation; (see parameters in Annex I.II.9.1.a) and Annex XIII of IVDR] will be specific issues before the more demanding tasks of **clinical evaluation** (CEV) of MD (under the CEV-plan; see chapter VI in this book) resp. **clinical performance evaluation** of IVDs (under the PEV[64]-Plan; see parameters of Annex I.II.9.1.b); see chapter VII in this book) will have to be undertaken. The relevant reports: clinical evaluation report (CER), see Tab. 13, resp. performance evaluation report (PER), see Tab. 18, are to be established and will be important parts of the **Technical Documentation**, demonstrating in detail overall conformity of the device and of important processes with the requirements of the applicable Regulation (see chapter X in this book and Annexes II and III (PMS) of the applicable Regulation).

Preparation for conformity assessment:

Pre-clarifications will have to focus on those mentioned in chapter XII.1 and XIII.1 (Qualification: does my device fall under MDR/IVDR? CE-marking or other specific route to market/user necessary [chapter XII.2 and XIII.2 in this book]? Which other EU/nat. legislation is applicable? Which class according

---

[63] See chapter 2 of this book
[64] PEV performance evaluation

to Annex VIII of Regulations?) The principal way to CE-marking is shown in Fig. 29.

Next consideration will be (if it is to go to CE-marking) which Annex/Annexes to choose[65] and the search for a suitable Notified Body (NB)[66] and the contract with it (see chapter XII.4 or XIII.4).

According to the Annex(es) chosen the relevant documentation (namely QMS-documentation, Technical documentation, Material for consultation procedures) has to be prepared; check for language requirements of NB!)

(initial) Conformity Assessment:

This will be done according to the choice of Annex(es) the manufacturer has taken according to the choices possible for the class of the device he has established following Annex VIII in both Regulations[67]; classes and related conformity assessment Annexes are correlated in MDR: Art. 52 for MD and in IVDR: Art. 48 for IVD[68]. Except for MD of class I (without Im, Is and Ir) and except for IVDs of class A non-sterile, where conformity assessment is to be done by the manufacturer on his own[69], conformity assessment is **performed by Notified Bodies (NBs)** acc. to Annexes IX – XI, as chosen. Additionally, in some kinds of high-risk devices an additional **consultation procedure[70]** is necessary (see MDR: Annex IX.5+6; Annex X.6; Annex XI.A.8+B.16; see IVDR: Annex IX.5. and Annex X.3.(j)+(k); Annex XI.5.; see chapter XII.7. and XIII.7. in this book). if the conformity assessment has been positively managed, the manufacturer has to collect and demonstrate the **signs of conformity**: CE marking of conformity (Annex V of MDR/IVDR), EU Declaration of Conformity (Annex IV of MDR/IVDR), certificate(s) of NB (Annex XII of MDR/IVDR), identification no. of NB.

---

[65] The possible choices for Annex(es) for each class are explained in MDR: Art. 52 resp. IVDR: Art. 48

[66] Theoretically 2 different NBs could be chosen, e.g. for Annex X and Annex XI

[67] see also chapter 11 in this book

[68] see chapter 12.6 for classes I – III for MD and chapter 13.6 for classes A – D for IVDs in this book

[69] Here manufacturers are only under market surveillance by their Competent Authorities

[70] Partly as batch testing in specific cases; see chapter 12.7 and 13.7 in this book

Conformity assessment will be followed by fulfilling the **registration requirements** according to Chapter III and Annex VI of both Regulations to the new European database **EUDAMED** and applying **UDI** (see Chapter III and Annex VI in both Regulations; chapter I.6. and IV in this book)

Post market:

EU Conformity assessment is not a single shot but the initial one is followed by **regular audits of the QMS** (at least annually, additionally unannounced ones are possible[71]). **Repetitions of representative assessments of technical documentations** will follow for the medium classes of devices[72]. PMS and Vigilance reporting is regularly observed by NBs, the higher the class, the more intense. **Change management** (planned changes of device, intended purpose and/or QMS; changes of harmonized standards or CS supplying presumptions of conformity and later changes of classification of devices) will be an important issue post market, often to be clarified and managed together with the NB.

Information on the quality, safety and performance of devices has to be systematically and pro-actively collected and analysed by the manufacturer and conclusions be drawn on improvements, updating of documentation, initiation and monitoring of corrective and preventive action and on reporting in the **PMS-system, based on a PMS-plan[73]**. The tip of the iceberg of this system is the **vigilance system[74]**, where serious incidents and field safety corrective actions (FSCA) will have to be reported to EUDAMED and urgently managed by the manufacturer to prevent similar incidents and risks to occur again. This will be done under close supervision by Member States.

Throughout the life cycle of a device the general obligations of the manufacturer will continue to apply[75].

---

[71] At least all 5 years

[72] See MDCG 2019-13: Guidance on sampling of devices for the assessment of the technical documentation

[73] Chapter 7.1 and Annex III of both Regulations; see chapter 15 in this book

[74] Chapter 7.2 in both Regulations; see chapter XVI in this book

[75] See Art. 10 of both Regulations; see chapter 3.1 in this book

Tab. 2 Overview Regulatory Compliance for MDR/IVDR

	Phase	Core elements	Main activities and challenges	Source in MDR/IVDR	Chapt. in this book
QMS	System	**QMS and Life-Cycle-(LC) Processes**	establish, document, implement, maintain, update, improve QMS with integrated LC processes (regulatory Compliance; RMS; CEV/PEV[76]; with resp. plans; Vigilance; Registration) poss. + processes: Software-Validation; Usability; etc	Art. 10; Annex IX+XI.A	3.1 + 12.5+6 MDR; 13.5+6 IVDR
	Premarket	**Qualification (delineation)**	Product falls under MDR/IVDR? Other EU/nat legislation applicable? **screening of the full regulatory profile to fulfil**	Chap I;	2
		General Safety and Performance Requirements, incl. RMS, CEV/PEV	**Which apply? Which to fulfil with presumptions of conformity by HN and CS and which with justified alternative solutions?** Incl. RMS und CEV/PEV[77];	Ann. I + Chap.VI MD: +Ann. XIV; IVD: + Ann. XIII	5-9
		Technical Documentation (TD)	**Draw-up and update TD** acc. Annex II + PMS-Plan acc. Annex III	Annex II+III	10+15

---

[76] Abbreviations see abbreviation list
[77] See fig. 11 - 14

Conformity Assessment – Market Access	Planning of market access	**Pre-clarifications**: Qualification? CE or other way? Classification? Choice of module(s)? choice of NB?	Chap I; Chap V;	2; 11; 12.1-4; 13.1-4;
		Conformity Assessment	application+documentation; acc. to module(s): IX: Audits + surveillance of QMS; assessment of TD (partly representastive);X: type examination+Ann.XI; poss. + consultation procedure	Ann IX-XI	12 + 13
		Proofs of conformity	Collect/draw-up: NB-certificate(s); CE-marking; 4-digit identification no of NB; EU-Declaration of Conformity;	Art 19/17; 20/18; Ann. IV, V	1.2.4.
		Registration	Registrations in EUDAMED; UDI	Chapt. III Ann. VI	4
		General MF obligations	QMS, LC-processes etc	Art. 10	3.1
Post-Market		**PMS-System**	PMS-System based on PMS-Plan; PMS-Reports; PSURs; draw conclusions, poss. CAPA, FSCA	Chap. VII.1 Ann. III	15
		Vigilance	Reports; protective measures, poss. CAPA, FSCA	Chap. VII.2	16
		LC-Processes	CEV-PMCF/PEV-PMPF; PMS; Vigilance; RMS	Ann XIV/XIII; Chapt VII; Annex I	5; 6; 7; 15; 16
		Surveillance by NB and CA	Surveillance audits; further assessment of TDs on random checks; NB receives and assesses PMS- and Vigilance reports; market surveillance by CAs	IX-XI; Chapt. VII.1-3	12+13; 15, 16

		Change management	In cooperation with NB: (planned) changes to device, intended purpose a/o QMS; changes to HS and CS, which deliver presumptions of conformity; changes to classification	Ann. IX-XI	12, 13

1.6. Transitional Provisions, Entry Into Force and Date of Application of MDR/IVDR

Main legal sources:

MDR: mainly Art. 120 - 123; as amended by REGULATION (EU) 2020/561;

IVDR: mainly Art. 110-113; as amended by REGULATION (EU) 2022/112

For the date of application of the MDR, pay special attention to REGULATION (EU) 2020/561 OF THE EUROPEAN PARLIAMENT AND OF THE COUNCIL of 23 April 2020 amending Regulation (EU) 2017/745 concerning medical devices, which **postponed the date of application of the MDR by 1 year, to 26.5.2021**!

Guidelines:

MDCG 2020-2 rev. 1: Class I transitional provisions under Article 120 (3 and 4) - (MDR);

MDCG 2020-3: Guidance on significant changes regarding the transitional provision under Article 120 of the MDR with regard to devices covered by certificates according to MDD or AIMDD.

[CAMD FAQ[78]: CAMD MDR/IVDR Transition Subgroup: FAQ – MDR Transitional provisions, is of Jan 2018 and therefore not necessarily up to date!]

---

[78] CAMD FAQ: Frequently asked questions by the Competent Authorities for Medical Devices, see https://www.camd-europe.eu/

Most important framework data of MDR/IVDR for the transitional phases (see Tab. 3)[79]:

Tab. 3 Transition regime of MDR/IVDR

	MDR, (resp. MDD/AIMDD)	**IVDR**, (resp. IVDD)
Publication in Official Journal of EU	05 May 2017	05 May 2017
Entry into Force (EiF)	25 May 2017	25 May 2017
New provisions for NB[80] from	26 Nov. 2017	26 Nov. 2017
Date of Application, DoA	26 May 2021[81] (4 years)	26 May 2022 (5 years)
End date of device to be in distribution chain[82] based on old NB certificate according to Directive	26 May 2025	See text below for IVD transition
NB certificate under Directive, issued before Entry into Force of relevant Regulation[83]:	„old" Certificate valid as indicated on it; except those for Annex 4/IV of the Directives, which will become void	„old" Certificate valid as indicated on it; except those for Annex VI of Directive, which will become void at

---

[79] Abbreviations used: MDD: Medical Device Directive = Directive 93/42/EEC; AIMDD: Active Implantable Medical Device Directive = Directive 90/385/EEC; IVDD: In vitro Diagnostics Directive = Directive 98/79/EC; EiF: Entry into Force; DoA: Date of Application; SAE: Serious Adverse Event; DD: Device Deficiency

[80] For those NBs, who have applied according to MDR: Art. 38 resp. IVDR: Art. 34; see current state of play: https://ec.europa.eu/docsroom/documents/32026

[81] acc. to REGULATION (EU) 2020/561 OF THE EUROPEAN PARLIAMENT AND OF THE COUNCIL of 23 April 2020 amending Regulation (EU) 2017/745 on medical devices, as regards the dates of application of certain of its provisions

[82] Making available or putting into service of device possible until this date, if (individual!) device has been lawfully placed on the market before DoA or after DoA based on a valid NB certificate (see lines of table below) under the relevant Directive (see MDR: Art. 120(4); IVDR: Art.110(4))

[83] Usually these certificates have a validity of 5 years; note that for devices placed on the market after DoA of MDR under these „old" certificates, they have still to comply with the provisions of the Directive, but no significant change in the design and intended purpose is possible and PMS, vigilance, market surveillance and registration provisions (if functional) of the MDR/IVDR apply.(MDR: Art. 120 (3); IVDR: Art. 110 (3))

	at the latest on 27 May 2022	the latest on 27 May 2025
Certificates under Directives, issued between EiF and DoA of Regulation[84]	max validity 5 years, but become void at the latest on 27 May 2024	become void at the latest on 27 May 2025
Clinical investigation resp. performance study starting before DoA	continue acc. to Directive, but SAE/DD-notifications acc. to MDR after DoA	continue acc. to Directive, but SAE/DD-notifications acc. to IVDR after DoA
Clinical investigation of MD/Performance study of IVD under multi-state procedure[85]	MDR: Between DoA and May 26, 2027: voluntary participation for MS concerned; then: mandatory participation at request of sponsor	IVDR: Between DoA and May 26, 2029: voluntary participation for MS concerned; then: mandatory participation at request of sponsor

MDR transition regime:

MDR: MDs that comply with the Regulation could be placed on the market before its date of application (May 26, 2021 for MDR) (for NB-certified products, only if suitable NBs newly designated under the Regulations are available and used[86]).

IVDR: see text below.

However, please note:

for MDR: <u>MDs that do not require certificates from NBs for conformity assessment according to the new regulation</u> (these would be: MDR: Class I, ex-

---

[84] Usually these certificates have a validity of 5 years; note that for devices placed on the market after DoA of MDR under these „old" certificates, they have still to comply with the provisions of the Directive, but no significant change in the design and intended purpose is possible and PMS, vigilance, market surveillance and registration provisions for actors and products (if functional) of the MDR/IVDR apply. (MDR: Art. 120 (3); IVDR: Art. 110 (3))

[85] Also called coordinated procedure, see chapters 8 and 9

[86] and some other requirements, e.g. existence of EU reference labs, expert panels, MDCG ready

cept classes Is, Im, Ir; and their manufacturers must comply with the requirements of MDR for placing on the market and putting into service as of the date of application of the regulation!

Extended validity of conformity assessment under Directive 93/42/EEC or Directive 90/385/EEC for certain MD with MDD/AIMDD certificates:

MDR: "Art 120 *(2) Certificates issued by notified bodies in accordance with Directives 90/385/EEC and 93/42/EEC prior to 25 May 2017 shall remain valid until the end of the period indicated on the certificate, except for certificates issued in accordance with Annex 4 to Directive 90/385/EEC or Annex IV to Directive 93/42/EEC which shall become void at the latest on 27 May 2022.*

Certificates issued by notified bodies in accordance with Directives 90/385/EEC and 93/42/EEC from 25 May 2017 shall remain valid until the end of the period indicated on the certificate, which shall not exceed five years from its issuance. They shall however become void at the latest on 27 May 2024."

The new text of Art. 120 (3) according to the amending Regulation (EU) 2020/561 to the MDR reads to this effect:

"(3) By way of derogation from Article 5 of this Regulation, a device which is a class I device pursuant to Directive 93/42/EEC, for which the declaration of conformity was drawn up prior to 26 May 2021 and for which the conformity assessment procedure pursuant to this Regulation requires the involvement of a notified body, or which has a certificate that was issued in accordance with Directive 90/385/EEC or Directive 93/42/EEC and that is valid by virtue of paragraph 2 of this Article, may be placed on the market or put into service until 26 May 2024, provided that from 26 May 2021 it continues to comply with either of those Directives, and provided there are no significant changes in the design and intended purpose. However, the requirements of this Regulation [means the MDR, the author] relating to post-market surveillance, market surveillance, vigilance, registration of economic operators and of devices shall apply in place of the corresponding requirements in those Directives.

Without prejudice to Chapter IV and paragraph 1 of this Article, the notified body that issued the certificate referred to in the first subparagraph shall continue to be responsible for the appropriate surveillance in respect of all of the applicable requirements relating to the devices it has certified."

The above mentioned Class I MDs of the Directive 93/42/EEC (without need of NB; but under MDR needing a NB) may in particular concern certain:

- MDs consisting of substances,
- MDs with nanomaterials,
- MD software,
- reusable surgical instruments of class I,
- inhalers,

for which these conditions may apply, as for these, a higher classification under the MDR and/or subsequently now the necessity of a NB may be possible[87]. For these devices *MDCG 2020-2 rev. 1: Class I transitional provisions under Article 120 (3 and 4) - (MDR)* will be helpful.

Please check the new text of Art. 120 (3) according to the amending Regulation (EU) 2020/561 to the MDR in this context, see above.

---

[87] You will have to check in each individual case!

Fig. 8 MDR Transitional Provisions

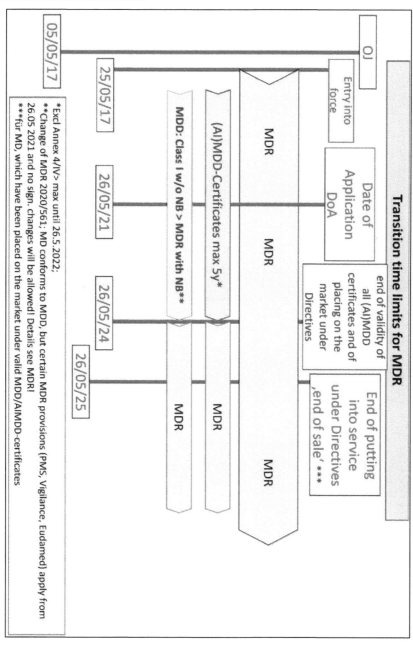

Transition time limits for MDR

| OJ | Entry into force | Date of Application DoA | end of validity of all (AI)MDD certificates and of placing on the market under Directives | End of putting into service under Directives ,end of sale'*** |

05/05/17

25/05/17

26/05/21

26/05/24

26/05/25

MDR

(AI)MDD-Certificates max 5y*

MDD: Class I w/o NB > MDR with NB**

* Excl Annex 4/IV> max until 26.5.2022;
**Change of MDR 2020/561; MD conforms to MDD, but certain MDR provisions (PMS, Vigilance, Eudamed) apply from 26.05 2021 and no sign. changes will be allowed! Details see MDR!
***für MD, which have been placed on the market under valid MDD/AIMDD-certificates

Fig. 9 IVDR Transitional Provisions (see detailed explanation below!)

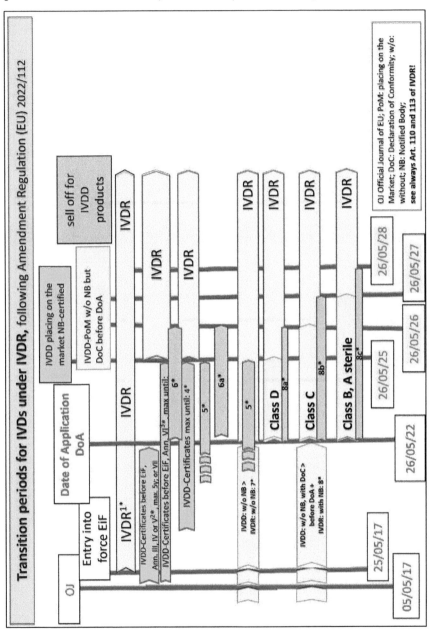

IVDR transition regime: See Fig.9 and the following explanations to Fig. 9 (please also look specifically at consolidated text of IVDR after Amendment Regulation (EU) 2022/112 [also below] and relevant MDCG documents):

Transitional provisions for IVDR follow 3 possible scenarios, see Fig.9:

A) Start immediately with IVDR:

1*: Placing on the market already possible under IVDR after Entry into Force (EiF) of IVDR, if IVD is IVDR-compliant; if NB needed, however additional conditions (e.g. suitable NBs must have been designated under IVDR [theoretically started 27 Nov 2017] and competent for that kind of IVD and its conformity assessment [codes and Annexes, see NANDO-system]; for high risk IVDs also MDCG, expert panels and EU ref labs had to be established; but look at some transitional provisions in MDCG 2021-4 Application of transitional provisions for certification of class D in vitro diagnostic medical devices according to Regulation (EU) 2017/746) and MDCG 2021-22: Clarification on "first certification for that type of device" and corresponding procedures to be followed by notified bodies, in context of the consultation of the expert panel referred to in Article 48(6) of Regulation (EU) 2017/746;

B) IVD has/had NB certificate under IVDD:

2*: IVDD certificates (except Annex VI), issued before entry into force of IVDR: valid as indicated on certificate (for Ann. III-V; i.e. max 5y acc. to IVDD, (which means expired before DoA of IVDR, unless prolonged before DoA of IVDR, see then 4*; wording of Art. 110 (3), 2nd subpara is somewhat ambiguous here!), Ann. VII certificates under IVDD-text not formally limited, but only applicable together with valid Annex V under IVDD; details see IVDR: Art. 110 (2), 1st subpara;

3*: Ann. VI [EC-Verification] certificates of IVDD, issued before entry into force of IVDR: here max validity until 26.5.2025; details see IVDR: Art. 110 (2), 1st subpara; please note, that Annex VI will only be applicable together with a valid Ann. V certificate under the IVDD;

4*: IVDD certificates, issued after entry into force but before DoA (Date of Application) of IVDR: valid until 26.05.2025; see Art. 110 (2), 2nd subpara;

5*: IVDs placed on the market following IVDD before DoA (Date of Application) of IVDR may be made available or put into service until 26.05.2025; see Art. 113 (4), 1st subpara;

6a*: IVDs placed on the market after DoA (Date of Application) of IVDR acc. to Art. 110 (2) [means IVDD certificate with prolonged validity according to Art. 110 (2)], may be made available or put into service until 26.05.2026 ('sell off'); see Art. 110 (4) 2nd subpara;

C) IVDs without necessity of IVDD NB-certificates:
7*IVDs without necessity of NB under IVDD and also none under IVDR (=Class A non sterile); at the latest at DoA (Date of Application) of IVDR: all IVDR-Requirements to be fulfilled, when placing on the market
8*IVDs placed on the market without necessity of NB-certification, but with DoC issued under IVDD (and other IVDD obligations) before DoA (Date of Application) of IVDR and which would now need a NB-certification under IVDR, may be placed on the market following IVDD until: [see Art. 110 (3), 3rd subpara; the corresponding sell off limits: see Art 110 (4), 2nd subpara]

> if Class D under IVDR: placing on the market under IVDD max until 26.05.2025, sell off of these IVDs placed on the market within that time period: max until 26.05.2026 (8a*);

> if Class C under IVDR: placing on the market under IVDD max until 26.05.2026, sell off of these IVDs placed on the market within that time period: max until 26.05.2027 (8b*);

> if Class B or Class A sterile under IVDR: placing on the market under IVDD max until 26.05.2027, sell off of these IVDs placed on the market within that time period: max until 26.05.2028 (8c*):

IVDs, placed on the market under IVDD, from DoA (Date of Application) of IVDR must still be in conformity with IVDD and, if applicable, under surveillance by IVDD-NB (see by analogy MDCG 2022-4); certain parts of IVDR will already be applicable from DoA (Date of Application) of IVDR (PMS, Vigilance, Eudamed [actor and product registration], market surveillance) and no sign. changes to design and intended purpose are possible!
Please always have a close look at IVDR: Art. 110 and 113!

See here the relevant text of the IVDR, consolidated version, after Amendment Regulation (EU) 2022/112, Art. 110:

2. Certificates issued by notified bodies in accordance with Directive 98/79/EC prior to 25 May 2017 shall remain valid until the end of the period indicated on the certificate, except for certificates issued in accordance with Annex VI to Directive 98/79/EC which shall become void at the latest on 27 May 2025.

Certificates issued by notified bodies in accordance with Directive 98/79/EC from 25 May 2017 shall become void by 27 May 2025.

3. By way of derogation from Article 5 of this Regulation, the devices referred to in the second and third subparagraphs of this paragraph may be placed on the market or put into service until the dates set out in those subparagraphs, provided that, from the date of application of this

Regulation, those devices continue to comply with Directive 98/79/EC, and provided that there are no significant changes in the design and intended purpose of those devices.

Devices with a certificate that was issued in accordance with Directive 98/79/EC and which is valid by virtue of paragraph 2 of this Article may be placed on the market or put into service until 26 May 2025.

Devices for which the conformity assessment procedure pursuant to Directive 98/79/EC did not require the involvement of a notified body, for which a declaration of conformity was drawn up prior to 26 May 2022 in accordance with that Directive, and for which the conformity assessment procedure pursuant to this Regulation requires the involvement of a notified body, may be placed on the market or put into service until the following dates:

(a) 26 May 2025, for class D devices;

(b) 26 May 2026, for class C devices;

(c) 26 May 2027, for class B devices;

(d) 26 May 2027, for class A devices placed on the market in sterile condition.

By way of derogation from the first subparagraph of this paragraph, the requirements of this Regulation relating to post-market surveillance, market surveillance, vigilance, registration of economic operators and of devices shall apply to devices referred to in the second and third subparagraphs of this paragraph instead of the corresponding requirements in Directive 98/79/EC.

Without prejudice to Chapter IV and paragraph 1 of this Article, the notified body that issued the certificate referred to in the second subparagraph of this paragraph shall continue to be responsible for the appropriate surveillance in respect of all applicable requirements relating to the devices it has certified.

4. Devices lawfully placed on the market pursuant to Directive 98/79/EC prior to 26 May 2022 may continue to be made available on the market or put into service until 26 May 2025.

Devices lawfully placed on the market from 26 May 2022 pursuant to paragraph 3 of this Article may continue to be made available on the market or put into service until the following dates:

(a) 26 May 2026 for devices referred to in paragraph 3, second subparagraph, or in paragraph 3, third subparagraph, point (a);

(b) 26 May 2027 for devices referred to in paragraph 3, third subparagraph, point (b);
(c) 26 May 2028 for devices referred to in paragraph 3, third subparagraph, points (c) and (d).';

Sell-off period for MDs:

The further making available or putting into service of **MDs** (= "sell-off from the trade chain") lawfully placed on the market before the date of application of the MDR (26.5.2021) according to MDD or AIMDD and those placed on the market after 26.5.2021 according to MDR: Art. 120 (3) is regulated in MDR: Art. 120 (4):

"(4) Devices lawfully placed on the market pursuant to Directives 90/385/EEC and 93/42/EEC prior to 26 May 2021, and devices placed on the market from 26 May 2021 pursuant to paragraph 3 of this Article, may continue to be made available on the market or put into service until 26 May 2025."

Sell-off periods for IVDs:

See above under transitional regime for IVDR, esp. IVDR: Art. 110 (4), which is repeated here:

4. Devices lawfully placed on the market pursuant to Directive 98/79/EC prior to 26 May 2022 may continue to be made available on the market or put into service until 26 May 2025.

Devices lawfully placed on the market from 26 May 2022 pursuant to paragraph 3 of this Article may continue to be made available on the market or put into service until the following dates:

(a) 26 May 2026 for devices referred to in paragraph 3, second subparagraph, or in paragraph 3, third subparagraph, point (a);
(b) 26 May 2027 for devices referred to in paragraph 3, third subparagraph, point (b);
(c) 26 May 2028 for devices referred to in paragraph 3, third subparagraph, points (c) and (d).';

Second Hand-Sales, within the EU only, are not affected by the Regulations[88].

---

[88] See recital (3) of both Regulations: This Regulation does not seek to harmonize rules relating to the further making available on the market of medical devices after they have already been put into service *[in the EU!! Remark by author]* such as in the context of second-hand

Exemptions granted by Member States under the previous Directives remain valid according to the conditions contained therein.

Provisions for the **new European database EUDAMED**[89] (see also chapter IV.1. in this book):

The provisions on the new EUDAMED database in principle will not enter into force until an independent audit has shown its overall functionality according to the specifications given by the COM in Cooperation with MDCG and the COM has published a communication to that effect in the Official Journal of the European Union (OJEU). As the regular date for the communication (25 March 2021) has been missed by the COM, EUDAMED (the modules for actors, Vigilance, Clinical Investigation&Performance Studies, and Market surveillance) would then become mandatory 6 months after such a delayed communication by the COM. The modules on UDI/Product registration and on NBs&Certificates become mandatory 24 months after the delayed Communication by the COM.

On a voluntary basis, the Commission has already deployed the **actor registration module as of 1 December 2020**. MDCG and Commission strongly encouraged the use of the actor registration module by all relevant actors on their territories, including the use of the single registration number by actors as stipulated in the MDR (for e.g. indicating the SRN on certificates). Also the **modules on product registration/UDI database** and the **module on NBs and their certificates** have already been activated in October 2021 on a voluntary basis.

The Independent Audit is currently foreseen for Q1/Q2 2023, the audit results will be discussed between COM and MDCG presumably Q2 2023; the Publication of a COM notice is planned for Q2 2023. End of 6 months after that Publication (Q4 2023) the modules for actors, Vigilance, Clinical Investigation&Performance Studies, and Market surveillance should become mandatory; at the end of 24 months after the Publication (Q2 2025) the modules

---

sales. See also Blue Guide of COM and chapter 1.3. of this book in this context. The regulations will however apply for second Hand-MDs/IVDs from 3rd countries imported into the EU.

[89] https://ec.europa.eu/health/medical-devices-eudamed/overview_en

on UDI/Product registration and on NBs&Certificates should become mandatory.

Please also note the **deadlines for the implementation of UDI carriers** according to MDR and IVDR, which are differentiated according to classes (in the case of MD also according to implantability): (see Tab. 4+5)[90]

Tab. 4 MDR: Time Limits for Application of UDI-Carriers

MD-Class /implantable?	Time limit	Reusable MD, when UDI-Carrier must be directly applied to the device (+ 2 years!)
implantable MD and Class III	26 May 2021	26 May 2023
Classes IIa and IIb, not implantable	26 May 2023	26 May 2025
Class I	26 May 2025	26 May 2027

Tab. 5 IVDR: Time Limits for Application of UDI-Carriers

IVD-Class	Time limit
Class D	26 May 2023
Classes B + C	26 May 2025
Class A	26 May 2027

---

[90] MDR: Art. 123.3. (f)+(g); IVDR: 113.3. (e)

Chapter 2. The Scope of the Two New Regulations: Product Delineation as a MD/IVD (Qualification)

Please note: Medical device is the overall term and includes IVDs as a sub-group of medical devices! However, the MDR only treats MDs that are not IVDs! The IVDR only treats IVDs[91]!

2.1 Does my product fall under the MDR?

Delineation of products as medical devices (Qualification)

Sources:

The main points you'll have to consider here are these sources of decision making:

Legally binding:

MDR: Chapter I, Art.1 with the inclusion and exclusion criteria and the fine-tuning of in-/exclusion, and Art. 2 with the relevant definitions, in particular those of the "medical device" and the "accessories for a medical device" and Art. 4 with the authorisation of the COM for implementing acts concerning delineations and Art. 23 (certain spare parts and components) and Art. 22 (systems and procedure packs) as well as Annex XVI (MD-like products without medical purpose, but with cosmetic or life-style purpose).

Important: when the MDR refers to "devices", it refers to MD, accessories for a MD or Annex XVI products[92]!

Implementing Acts of the COM acc. to Art. 4 of MDR (if any):

In addition to individual decisions by the member states on demarcation issues, the COM, on its own initiative or at the request of a member state, also has the option of deciding uniformly in individual cases whether a specific product or a specific category or group of products constitutes a "medical

---

[91] please note the possibility of integral MD-IVD combination products acc. to MDR: Art. 1 (7) and IVDR: Art. 1 (4): in this case both Regulations would apply, each for the corresponding part. A system or procedure pack acc. to MDR: Art. 22 may also include CE-marked MDs and CE-marked IVDs!

[92] Acc to MDR: Art. 1 (2)

device" or an "accessory for a medical device" by means of an implementing Act in accordance with Art. 4. Support in the preparation of such decisions can be provided by relevant EU agencies.

Finally, judgments of the **European Court of Justice (ECJ)** must also be observed, as the ECJ is authorised to make legally binding interpretations on EU law.

Guidelines (not legally binding, but esp. as MDCG[93] guidances highly recommended to be considered):

MDCG 2019-11: Qualification and classification of software - Regulation (EU) 2017/745 and Regulation (EU) 2017/746;

MEDDEV[94] 2.1/3 rev.3: Guidance document - Scope, field of application, definition - Borderline products, drug-delivery products and medical devices incorporating, as integral part, an ancillary medicinal substance or an ancillary human blood derivative – [still important for delineation towards pharmaceuticals! MDCG guideline in preparation]

MEDDEV 2.1/2 rev.2: Guidance document - Field of application of directive "active implantable medical devices" -

MEDDEV 2.1/2.1: Guidance document - Field of application of directive "active implantable medical devices" - Treatment of computers used to program implantable pulse generators –

Guidelines EMA

Please have the EMA's guidelines on your screen if you have to solve demarcation problems with the medicinal product sector. They are also helpful for the treatment of ancillary medicinal product components of your MD[95] or in case of certain substances/substance combinations and the associated consultation procedures in conformity assessment with medicinal product authorities in the EU:

---

[93] MDCG Medical Device Coordination Group of the EU

[94] MEDDEVs are formally interpreting the medical device directives and will have to be adjusted to MDR/IVDR; sometimes they may still be useful for the MDR/IVDR, if the text of MDR/IVDR is not substantially differing

[95] E.g. a drug eluting coronary stent

https://www.ema.europa.eu/en/human-regulatory/overview/medical-devices

The **scope of the MDR** with inclusion and exclusion criteria of the MDR is shown in Fig. 10.

Important: please have a look both at inclusion <u>and</u> exclusion criteria of the MDR and consider some fine-tuning for specific problem-zones for qualification, where a closer look will be necessary, namely for:

- o medicinal products (pharmaceuticals);
- o biological components of human, animal or microorganismic origin;
- o software;

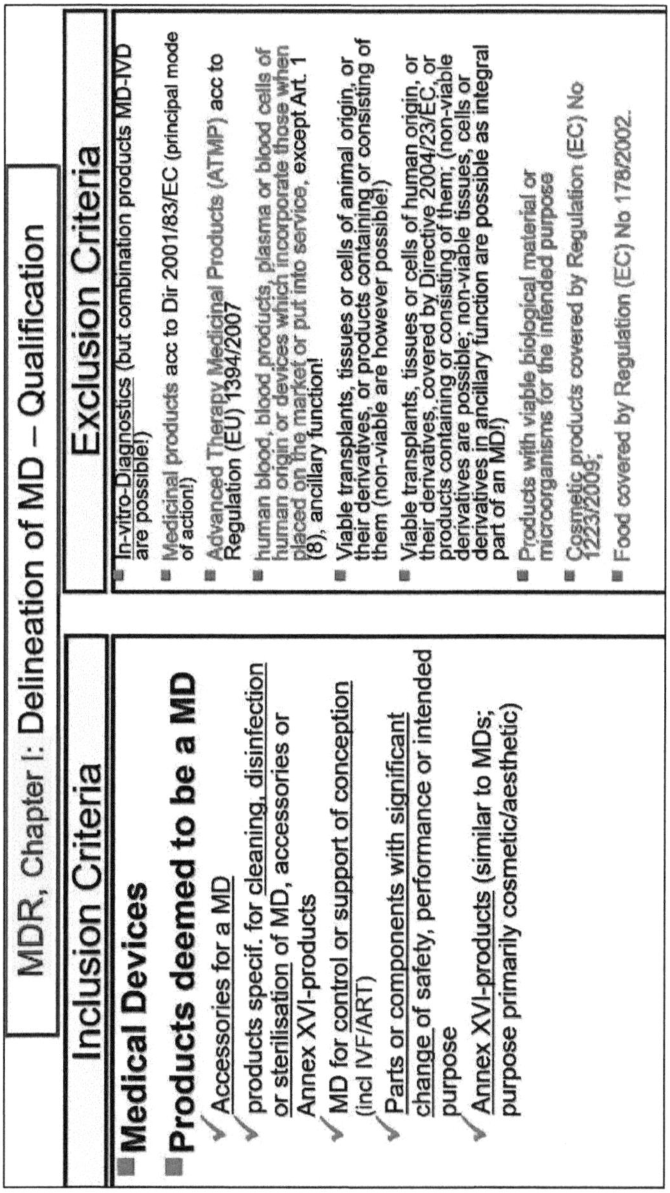

Fig. 10 MDR: Delineation Overview

MDR, Chapter I: Delineation of MD – Qualification

Inclusion Criteria	Exclusion Criteria

■ **Medical Devices**
 	
■ **Products deemed to be a MD**
  ✓ Accessories for a MD
  ✓ products specif. for cleaning, disinfection or sterilisation of MD, accessories or Annex XVI-products
  ✓ MD for control or support of conception (incl IVF/ART)
  ✓ Parts or components with significant change of safety, performance or intended purpose
  ✓ Annex XVI-products (similar to MDs; purpose primarily cosmetic/aesthetic)
	■ In-vitro-Diagnostics (but combination products MD-IVD are possible!)
	■ Medicinal products acc to Dir 2001/83/EC (principal mode of action!)
	■ Advanced Therapy Medicinal Products (ATMP) acc to Regulation (EU) 1394/2007
	■ human blood, blood products, plasma or blood cells of human origin or devices which incorporate those when placed on the market or put into service, except Art. 1 (8), ancillary function!
	■ Viable transplants, tissues or cells of animal origin, or their derivatives, or products containing or consisting of them (non-viable are however possible!)
	■ Viable transplants, tissues or cells of human origin, or their derivatives, covered by Directive 2004/23/EC, or products containing or consisting of them; (non-viable derivatives are possible; non-viable tissues, cells or derivatives in ancillary function are possible as integral part of an MD!)
	■ Products with viable biological material or microorganisms for the intended purpose
	■ Cosmetic products covered by Regulation (EC) No 1223/2009;
	■ Food covered by Regulation (EC) No 178/2002.

A **systematic examination procedure** to determine whether a product falls under the MDR can therefore be performed as follows (for manufacturers under the QMS!; please note again, that both the inclusion and exclusion criteria will have to be examined):

Step I: Check whether the product falls under the definition of a "medical device" or of a "product deemed to be a medical device"
(= check for inclusion criteria):

I.A) Check whether the definition "medical device" applies.

I.B) Examination as to whether the product falls under "a product deemed to be a medical device[96]":

Let's look at this now in more detail:

1A) Check whether the definition "medical device" applies:

Look at the MDR's definition of MD, here separated into 3 parts:

---

*MDR: Art. 2 (1): '**medical device**' means any instrument, apparatus, appliance, software, implant, reagent, material or other article intended by the manufacturer to be used, alone or in combination,*

--

for human beings for one or more of the following specific medical purposes:
— diagnosis, prevention, monitoring, prediction, prognosis, treatment or alleviation of disease,
— diagnosis, monitoring, treatment, alleviation of, or compensation for, an injury or disability,
— investigation, replacement or modification of the anatomy or of a physiological or pathological process or state,
— providing information by means of in vitro examination of specimens derived from the human body, including organ, blood and tissue donations,

--

and which does not achieve its principal intended action by pharmacological, immunological or metabolic means, in or on the human body, but which may be assisted in its function by such means.

The first part of the definition points to the kinds of entities, which in principle may qualify for a medical device; this is a really broad range!

The 2nd part deals with a broad overview of the specific medical purposes to be achieved by medical devices. This part is kept very general; for any specific MD this must be highly specified by the manufacturer with regard to specific diseases (incl. stages, severities etc.) to be targeted and the corresponding target (patient) groups, where the device is intended to achieve its clinical performance and clinical benefit. See the details needed to establish the intended purpose of a MD in chapter X of this book.

The 3rd part of the definition tries to distinguish between pharmaceuticals (medicinal products) and medical devices with a reference to the principal intended action of the product in question. The principal mode of action of pharmaceuticals is based on pharmaceutical, immunological or metabolic means[97], whereas the mode of action of medical devices usually is a physical/physicalistic one. The principal mode of action of the product must be underpinned by the manufacturer with a scientific rationale and proof.

---

[97] these means are explained in the MEDDEV 2.1/3 rev 3 on delineation of MD and pharmaceuticals [a MDCG guidance on these means is in preparation]:

"Pharmacological means" is understood as an interaction between the molecules of the substance in question and a cellular constituent, usually referred to as a receptor, which either results in a direct response, or which blocks the response to another agent. Although not a completely reliable criterion, the presence of a dose-response correlation is indicative of a pharmacological effect.

"Immunological means" is understood as an action in or on the body by stimulation and/or mobilisation of cells and/or products involved in a specific immune reaction.

"Metabolic means" is understood as an action which involves an alteration, including stopping, starting or changing the speed of the normal chemical processes participating in, and available for, normal body function.

Note: The fact that a product is, or is not, itself metabolised does not imply that it achieves, or does not achieve, its principal intended action by metabolic means.

Medical devices may be assisted in their function by pharmacological, immunological or metabolic means, but as soon as these means are not ancillary with respect to the principal intended action of a product, the product no longer fulfils the definition of a medical device. The claims made for a product, in accordance with its method of action may, in this context, represent an important factor for its qualification as a medical device. These principles can be, for example, illustrated by bone cements. Plain bone cement without antibiotics is a medical device since it achieves its principal intended action (the fixation of prosthesis) by physical means. Bone cements containing antibiotics, where the principal intended action remains fixation of prosthesis, are also medical devices. In this case the action of the antibiotic, which is to reduce the possibility of infection being introduced during surgery, is clearly ancillary. If

<u>1B) Examination as to whether the product falls under "a product deemed to be a medical device":</u>

- **Accessories for a medical device** (Art. 2 (2)):

'accessory for a medical device' means an article which, whilst not being itself a medical device, is intended by its manufacturer to be used together with one or several particular medical device(s) to specifically enable the medical device(s)

  - *to be used in accordance with its/their intended purpose(s) or*
  - *to specifically and directly assist the medical functionality of the medical device(s) in terms of its/their intended purpose(s);* [bullets edited by author for better comprehension]

- **devices for the control or support of conception**[98]:

- **products specifically intended for the cleaning, disinfection or sterilisation** of devices as referred to in Article 1(4) and of those referred to in the first paragraph of this point; (meaning medical devices, accessories, Annex XVI-products and devices for the control or support of conception). Major devices in that sector would be sterilizers (e.g. by moist heat, EO, radiation) and washer-disinfectors[99] (e.g. for endoscopes)

- **Parts or components** specially designed to replace a part or component of an MD and which significantly change its performance, safety or intended purpose; (MDR: Art. 23)

- **Annex XVI products** (MD-like products without medical purpose, but with cosmetic or lifestyle purpose, e.g. liposuction equipment, cosmetic implants or fillers), which are listed in Annex XVI of the MDR, as soon as common specifications (CS) apply to them; the list may in future be extended by the COM through delegated acts.

---

however the principal intended action is to deliver the antibiotic, the product no longer fulfils the definition of a medical device.

An MDCG Guidance on Borderline with medicinal products (including general guidance, definitions of pharmacological, immunological and metabolic means of action and diagnosis) is in preparation: https://ec.europa.eu/health/sites/health/files/md_sector/docs/mdcg_ongoing_guidancedocs_en.pdf . You should also have a look at EMA's (European Medicines Agency) guidance on the interface with medical devices: https://www.ema.europa.eu/en/human-regulatory/overview/medical-devices .

[98] For devices for support of conception see also: MEDDEV 2.2/4: Conformity assessment of in vitro fertilisation (IVF) and assisted reproduction technologies (ART) products, which has still to be adapted to MDR

[99] See EN ISO 15883-series

> **Step II: Examination for detailed exclusion criteria,** especially according to Art.1 of MDR, **and for fine-tuning of in-/exclusion:**

The MDR would not apply to (=Excluded are):

II.A) IVD covered by IVDR[100]

II.B) Medicinal products[101] (pharmaceuticals)

Please note in connection with **pharmaceuticals** (finetuning):

> a) Any device which, when placed on the market or put into service, incorporates, as an <u>integral part</u>[102], a substance which, if used separately, would be considered to be a medicinal product[103], and that has an <u>action ancillary</u> to that of the device, shall be assessed and authorised in accordance with MDR. (MDR: Art.1 (8), 1st subpara)
>
> b) However, <u>if the action of that substance is principal</u> and not ancillary to that of the device, the integral product shall be governed by Directive 2001/83/EC[104] or Regulation (EC) No 726/2004[105], as applicable. In that case, the relevant general safety and performance requirements set out in Annex I of MDR shall apply as far as the safety and

---

[100] But please note the possibility of integral MD-IVD combination products acc. to MDR: Art. 1 (7) and IVDR: Art. 1 (4): in this case both Regulations would apply, each for the corresponding part. CE-marked IVDs may also be part of systems or procedure packs acc. to MDR: Art. 22.

[101] medicinal products as defined in point 2 of Article 1 of Directive 2001/83/EC. In deciding whether a product falls under Directive 2001/83/EC or under MDR, particular account shall be taken of the principal mode of action of the product; a principal mode of action based on pharmaceutical, immunological or metabolic means would be considered as those of a pharmaceutical and these means are explained in the MEDDEV 2.1/3 rev 3 on delineation of MD and pharmaceuticals (see also 3rd part of the definition of a medical device, as above).

[102] MEDDEV 2.1/3 rev.3. B.4.: A medical device incorporates a medicinal substance as an <u>integral part</u>, within the meaning of Article 1 (4) MDD and Article 1 (4) AIMDD, if and only if the device and the substance are physically or chemically combined at the time of administration (i.e. use, implantation, application etc) to the patient.

[103] as defined in point 2 of Article 1 of Directive 2001/83/EC, including a medicinal product derived from human blood or human plasma as defined in point 10 of Article 1 of that Directive

[104] Directive 2001/83/EC of the European Parliament and of the Council of 6 November 2001 on the Community code relating to medicinal products for human use

[105] Regulation (EC) No 726/2004 of the European Parliament and of the Council of 31 March 2004 laying down Community procedures for the authorisation and supervision of medicinal products for human and veterinary use and establishing a European Medicines Agency

performance of the device part are concerned. (MDR: Art.1 (8), 2nd sub-para).

c) Any device which is intended to administer a medicinal product[106] shall be governed by MDR, without prejudice to the provisions of that Directive and of Regulation (EC) No 726/2004 with regard to the medicinal product. (MDR: Art.1 (9), 1st subpara).

d) However, if the device intended to administer a medicinal product and the medicinal product are placed on the market in such a way that they <u>form a single integral[107] product</u> which is <u>intended exclusively for use in the given combination and which is not reusable</u>, that single integral product shall be governed by Directive 2001/83/EC or Regulation (EC) No 726/2004, as applicable. In that case, the relevant general safety and performance requirements set out in Annex I of MDR shall apply as far as the safety and performance of the device part of the single integral product are concerned. (MDR: Art.1 (9), 2nd subpara)

e) see also MDR: Art. 22.1.c) on systems and procedure packs, where pharmaceuticals could now be part of such (medically meaningful) systems or procedure packs if in line with pharmaceutical legislation.

f) see also II.C and II.D below.

II.C) Advanced therapy medicinal products within the meaning of Regulation (EC) No 1394/2007[108],(ATMP);

II.D) human blood, blood products, plasma or blood cells of human origin or devices which incorporate, when placed on the market or put into service, such blood products, plasma or cells, except for devices referred to in paragraph 8 of this Article; (i.e. under II.B) (a) above; similar under II.B.(c) above);

---

[106] as defined in point 2 of Article 1 of Directive 2001/83/EC

[107] MEDDEV 2.1/3 rev.3. B.4.: A medical device incorporates a medicinal substance as an <u>integral part</u>, within the meaning of Article 1 (4) MDD and Article 1 (4) AIMDD, if and only if the device and the substance are physically or chemically combined at the time of administration (i.e. use, implantation, application etc) to the patient.

[108] Regulation (EC) No 1394/2007 of the European Parliament and of the Council of 13 November 2007 on advanced therapy medicinal products and amending Directive 2001/83/EC and Regulation (EC) No 726/2004. ATMP: Dealing with gene therapy, somatic cell therapy and tissue engineering.

II.E) **cosmetic products** within the meaning of Regulation (EC) No 1223/2009[109],

II.F) viable **transplants, tissues or cells of animal origin, or their derivatives**, or products containing or consisting of them, are also excluded from MDR; (however this Regulation *[=MDR]* does apply to devices manufactured utilising tissues or cells of animal origin, or their derivatives, which are non-viable or are rendered non-viable[110]);

II.G) **viable transplants, tissues or cells of human origin, or their derivatives**, covered by Directive 2004/23/EC[111], or products containing or consisting of them are also excluded from MDR; (however this Regulation *[=MDR]* does apply to devices manufactured utilising derivatives of tissues or cells of human origin which are non-viable or are rendered non-viable[112]);

Please note further for **components of human origin**:

a) Any device which, when placed on the market or put into service, incorporates, as an integral part, non-viable tissues or cells of human origin or their derivatives that have an action ancillary to that of the device shall be assessed and authorised in accordance with MDR. In that case, the provisions for donation, procurement and testing laid down in Directive 2004/23/EC shall apply. (MDR: Art.1 (10), 1st subpara)

b) However, if the action of those tissues or cells or their derivatives is principal and not ancillary to that of the device and the product is not governed by Regulation (EC) No 1394/2007, the product shall be governed by Directive 2004/23/EC. In that case, the relevant general safety and performance requirements set out in Annex I of MDR shall apply as far as the safety and performance of the device part are concerned. (MDR: Art.1 (10), 2nd subpara)

---

[109] Regulation (EC) No 1223/2009 of the European Parliament and of the Council of 30 November 2009 on cosmetic products

[110] MDR: Art.2 Nr. 16: non-viable' means having no potential for metabolism or multiplication

[111] Directive 2004/23/EC of the European Parliament and of the Council of 31 March 2004 on setting standards of quality and safety for the donation, procurement, testing, processing, preservation, storage and distribution of human tissues and cells.

[112] MDR: Art.2 Nr. 16: non-viable' means having no potential for metabolism or multiplication

II.H) **products** other than those referred to in points (d), (f) and (g) *[i.e. II.D, II.F and II.G above – the author]* which consist of or contain **viable biological material or viable organisms, including living micro-organisms, bacteria, fungi or viruses**, in order to achieve or support the intended purpose[113] of the product are also excluded from MDR;

II.I. **Food** as defined in Regulation (EC) No 178/2002.

II.J. Notes on the delineation of **software**:

Questions of qualification and classification of software as a medical device are discussed by a separate group of experts under the MDCG; results, which usually follow a **modular approach[114]**, can be found in "MDCG 2019-11: Qualification and classification of software - Regulation (EU) 2017/745 and Regulation (EU) 2017/746". In it's Chapters 3.2. and 3.3. 'Medical Device Software (MDSW)'[115] is distinguished from 'Software driving or influencing the use of a medical device'[116]. Figure 1 and 2 of this MDCG 2019-11 contain a number of decision steps (decision tree) for qualification of MDSW as either a medical device (Figure 1) or an in vitro diagnostic medical device (Figure 2)

Annex I of MDCG 2019-11: gives illustrative examples of qualification of

---

[113] The reference to intended purpose is important here, as otherwise all non-sterile MDs would have been excluded from the scope of the MDR!

[114] See specifically the MDCG 2019-11, chapter 7

[115] MDCG 2019-11: *Software: For the purpose of this guidance, "software" is defined as a set of instructions that processes input data and creates output data.*
Medical device software (MDSW) is software that is intended to be used, alone or in combination, for a purpose as specified in the definition of a "medical device" in the MDR or IVDR, regardless of whether the software is independent or driving or influencing the use of a device.

[116] *'Software driving or influencing the use of a medical device' is software intended to drive or influence the use of a (hardware)medical device and does not have or perform a medical purpose on its own, nor does it create information on its own for one or more of the medical purposes described in the definition of a medical device or an in vitro diagnostic medical device. This software can, but is not limited to:*
a) operate, modify the state of, or control the device either through an interface (e.g., software, hardware) or via the operator of this device
b) or supply output related to the (hardware) functioning of that device
Note: Software that is driving or influencing the use of a medical device is covered by the medical devices regulations either as a part/component of a device or as an accessory for a medical device.

software used in the healthcare environment; Annex II – gives Qualification examples of Medical Device Software (MDSW) according to Figures 1 and 2.

2.2 Does my product fall under the IVDR?

(Qualification of in vitro diagnostics)

2.2.1. Sources:

Where can you find the **legal basis for qualification in the IVDR?**

2.2.1.1. Legally binding documents:

You should pay particular attention to **IVDR Chapter I, Art.1** with the inclusion and exclusion criteria and **Art.2** with the relevant definitions, in particular those of the "medical device", the "in vitro diagnostic medical device" and the "accessory for an in vitro diagnostic medical device".

Important: When "devices" are mentioned in the IVDR, this means IVDs or accessories for an IVD!

For proper delineation (qualification) you have to look first for inclusion criteria, then to exclusion criteria of the IVDR, see the steps below.

IVDR: Art. 20 deals with specific parts and components, which might be deemed to be IVDs (if they would provide significant changes, see below)

Additional legally binding decisions/documents under the IVDR or national legislation:

Art.3 includes the **authorization of the COM for implementing acts concerning demarcations**, so you should be aware whether such implementing acts exist:

The COM, on its own initiative or at the request of a member state, must decide uniformly by implementing acts acc. to IVDR: Art. 3, whether a specific product or a specific category or group of products constitutes an IVD or an accessory for an IVD; support in the preparation of such decisions may be provided by relevant EU agencies.

Finally, **judgments of the European Court of Justice** (ECJ) must also be observed within the framework of its sovereignty of interpretation over EU law. In addition, but not in contradiction to the above, **decisions by the member states (administrative or judicial by local courts) on qualification issues** are possible and you should have them on your screen.

2.2.1.2. Non-legally binding interpretative documents:

The primary source of such guidance under the IVDR is now **MDCG, the Medical Device Coordination Group[117]**:

MDCG 2019-11: Qualification and classification of software - Regulation (EU) 2017/745 and Regulation (EU) 2017/746.

Another source of guidance may be **CAMD, the EU Competent Authorities for Medical Devices** (and IVDs)[118].

Older guidance (for the IVDD) have been provided by the COM as **MEDDEVs** (Medical Device Guidelines) which have been prepared jointly with the stakeholders. These may still provide assistance with questions of qualification, especially MEDDEVs 2.14/1 (Borderline and classification[119] of IVDs) and /2 (Research use only products) and the **Manual** (with individual "decisions" supported by involved stakeholders), but which still need to be adapted to the IVDR in form and, if necessary, in content. So when relying on these MEDDEVs and the Manual you have to be careful, which interpretations of the IVDD may be transferred to the IVDR.

European decisions and interpretative documents, like MDCG guidance and MEDDEVs, Manuals etc are offered on the COM homepage of the MD/IVD sector (see link list); there are also useful links to relevant legislation/decisions/guidelines in other sectors.

National competent authorities may also provide guidance.

Changes to regulations, creation of relevant new implementing or delegated acts or changes to those, or new legally binding opinions or judgments of the ECJ as well as creation of new or changes to non-legally binding documents (e.g. MDCG guidances) concerning delineation will have to be anticipated

---

[117] See MDCG guidance and planned guidance under: https://ec.europa.eu/health/md_sector/new_regulations/guidance_en

[118] https://www.camd-europe.eu/

[119] May still be useful for some qualification issues, but completely outdated for classification issues!

and monitored by the manufacturer in his **change management under his QMS**[120].

An Overview of IVD qualification with inclusion and exclusion criteria under the IVDR can be found in Fig. 11:

---

[120] There must be a process in place under the manufacturer's QMS to assure regulatory compliance when regulatory or interpretational changes are imminent (usually there are public consultation procedures before or newsletters of the COM or Competent Authorities or of stakeholder organisations announcing changes or information provided on their homepages) or are being implemented.

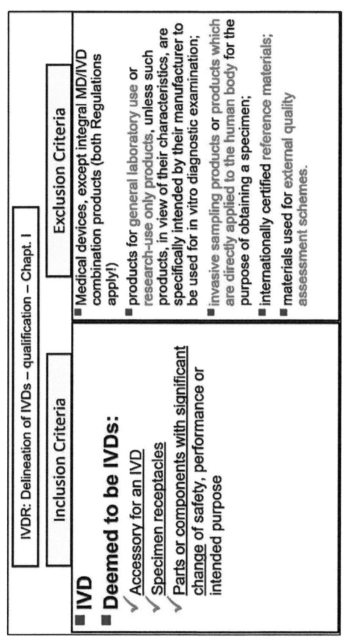

Fig. 11 IVDR: Delineation Overview

A systematic test procedure to determine whether a product falls under the IVDR can therefore be as follows (for manufacturers under the QMS! Please always look both at inclusion <u>and</u> exclusion criteria applying!):

> **Step I: Check whether the product falls under "IVD" or "product deemed to be an IVD" (= inclusion criteria):**

Check whether the product falls under the following definitions:

I.A) Does the product fall under the definition of an In vitro diagnostic medical device?

I.B) Does the product fall under a 'product deemed to be an IVD'?

I.A) Does it fall under an **In vitro diagnostic medical device?**,

> *IVDR: Art.2 (2): 'in vitro diagnostic medical device'*
> *means any medical device*
> --
> *which is a reagent, reagent product, calibrator, control material, kit, instrument, apparatus, piece of equipment, software or system, whether used alone or in combination,*
> --
> *intended by the manufacturer <u>to be used in vitro for the examination of specimens, including blood and tissue donations, derived from the human body,</u> solely or principally*
> --
> *for the purpose of providing information on one or more of the following:*
> *(a) concerning a physiological or pathological process or state;*
> *(b) concerning congenital physical or mental impairments;*
> *(c) concerning the predisposition to a medical condition or a disease;*
> *(d) to determine the safety and compatibility with potential recipients;*
> *(e) to predict treatment response or reactions;*
> *(f) to define or monitoring therapeutic measures.*
> --
> *Specimen receptacles shall also be deemed to be in vitro diagnostic medical devices;*

For a systematic examination approach, I have divided this definition of an IVD into 5 boxes:

The <u>first box</u> indicates, that an IVD must in any case be a medical device first, acc. to the definition of an MD given in IVDR: Art. 2 (1) relating to the definition of an MD in the MDR.

The <u>2nd box</u> refers to those kinds of entities, which in principle might fall under the definition of an IVD. The following definitions of the IVDR will help you here:

IVDR: Art. 2 (11): *'kit' means a set of components that are packaged together and intended to be used to perform a specific in vitro diagnostic examination, or a part thereof;*

IVDR: Art. 2 (55): *'calibrator' means a measurement reference material used in the calibration of a device;*

IVDR: Art. 2 (56): *'control material' means a substance, material or article intended by its manufacturer to be used to verify the performance characteristics of a device;*

With regard to **software**[121] as an IVD, please look at MDCG Guidance 2019-11: Qualification and classification of software - Regulation (EU) 2017/745 and Regulation (EU) 2017/746. In this MDCG guidance 'Medical Device Software (MDSW)' is distinguished from 'Software driving or influencing the use of a medical device' . Figure 1 and 2 of this MDCG 2019-11 contain a number of decision steps (decision tree) for qualification of MDSW as either a

---

[121] MDCG 2019-11: *Software: For the purpose of this guidance, "software" is defined as a set of instructions that processes input data and creates output data.*
Medical device software (MDSW) *is software that is intended to be used, alone or in combination, for a purpose as specified in the definition of a "medical device" in the MDR or IVDR, regardless of whether the software is independent or driving or influencing the use of a device.*
 'Software driving or influencing the use of a medical device' is software intended to drive or influence the use of a (hardware)medical device and does not have or perform a medical purpose on its own, nor does it create information on its own for one or more of the medical purposes described in the definition of a medical device or an in vitro diagnostic medical device. This software can, but is not limited to:
a) operate, modify the state of, or control the device either through an inter-face (e.g., software, hardware) or via the operator of this device
b) or supply output related to the (hardware) functioning of that device
Note: Software that is driving or influencing the use of a medical device is covered by the medical devices regulations either as a part/component of a device or as an accessory for a medical device.

medical device (Figure 1) or an in vitro diagnostic medical device (Figure 2)

Annex I of MDCG 2019-11: gives illustrative examples of qualification of software used in the healthcare environment; Annex II – gives Qualification examples of Medical Device Software (MDSW) according to Figures 1 and 2.

The 3rd box of the IVD definition within IVDR indicates 3 important elements of the definition of an IVD: as intended by the manufacturer, they are to be used in vitro and they are intended for the examination of specimens, including blood and tissue donations, derived from the human body, (not for veterinary purposes!) with the aim of providing hopefully medically useful and reliable information, which is further exemplified in the next box.

The 4th box contains the specific medical purposes where they are intended to provide (hopefully medically useful and reliable) information. At 2 points this definition has been specified against the one in the IVDD, namely c) with regard to medical genetic testing and e) to predict treatment response or reactions, which relates to companion diagnostics[122] and is important for personalized or precision medicine.

The 5th box indicates, that 'specimen receptacles' are deemed to be IVDs; see below under IB).

---

[122] *'companion diagnostic'* means a device which is essential for the safe and effective use of a corresponding medicinal product to:
(a) identify, before and/or during treatment, patients who are most likely to benefit from the corresponding medicinal product; or
(b) identify, before and/or during treatment, patients likely to be at increased risk of serious adverse reactions as a result of treatment with the corresponding medicinal product;
In this context, please have a look at recitals (11) and (12) of IVDR:
IVDR: Recitals: (11) Companion diagnostics are essential for defining patients' eligibility for specific treatment with a medicinal product through the quantitative or qualitative determination of specific markers identifying subjects at a higher risk of developing an adverse reaction to the medicinal product in question or identifying patients in the population for whom the therapeutic product has been adequately studied, and found safe and effective. Such biomarker or biomarkers can be present in healthy subjects and/or in patients.
(12) Devices that are used with a view to monitoring treatment with a medicinal product in order to ensure that the concentration of relevant substances in the human body is within the therapeutic window are not considered to be companion diagnostics.

I.B) Is it a **Product Deemed to be an IVD?** These might be:

- **Accessory for an in vitro diagnostic medical device**[123], IVDR: Art. 2 (4): *'accessory for an in vitro diagnostic medical device' means an article which, whilst not being itself an in vitro diagnostic medical device, is intended by its manufacturer to be used together with one or several particular in vitro diagnostic medical device(s)*
    - *to specifically enable the in vitro diagnostic medical device(s) to be used in accordance with its/their intended purpose(s) or*
    - *to specifically and directly assist the medical functionality of the in vitro diagnostic medical device(s) in terms of its/their intended purpose(s);*[124]
- **Specimen receptacles**[125], IVDR: Art. 2 (3): *'specimen receptacle' means a device, whether of a vacuum-type or not, specifically intended by its manufacturer for the primary containment and preservation of specimens derived from the human body for the purpose of in vitro diagnostic examination;*
- **Parts or components** specifically intended to replace a part or component of an IVD and <u>which significantly change its performance, safety or intended purpose</u>[126];

> **Step II: Checking for exclusion criteria and finetuning of in-/exclusion,**

especially according to Art.1. of IVDR.

The IVDR does not apply to (=exclusion criteria):

II.A. **Medical devices** within the meaning of MDR [which are not IVDs], but the IVDR applies to the IVD part of integral MD-IVD combination products[127];

---

[123] See here IVDR: Art.1. 2. *For the purposes of this Regulation, in vitro diagnostic medical devices and accessories for in vitro diagnostic medical devices shall hereinafter be referred to as 'devices'.*

[124] [bullets introduced by author for better understanding]

[125] see also MEDDEV 2.14/1 rev 2 chapter 1.3. for examples under the IVDD [alignment with IVDR still necessary!]

[126] IVDR: Art. 20.2.

[127] see IVDR: Art.1 (4) and MDR: Art. 1 (7). Both Regulations would apply, each to its specific part. IVDR: Art.1.4: *4. Any device which, when placed on the market or put into service, incorporates, as an integral part, a medical device as defined in point 1 of Article 2 of Regulation*

II.B. **Products for general laboratory use**[128], unless such products, in view of their characteristics, are specifically intended by their manufacturer to be used for in vitro diagnostic examination;

II.C. **Products intended for research purposes only**[129], unless such products, in view of their characteristics, are specifically intended by their manufacturer to be used for in vitro diagnostic examination;

II.D. **invasive sampling products or products which are directly applied to the human body for the purpose of obtaining a specimen**[130];

II.E. **internationally certified reference materials**;

II.F. **Materials for external quality evaluation programs**.

(EU) 2017/745 [=MDR] *shall be governed by that Regulation. The requirements of this Regulation* [=IVDR] *shall apply to the in vitro diagnostic medical device part.*

[128] See here specifically MEDDEV 2.14/1 rev 2, chapter 1.4 with examples [the MEDDEV has to be formally and in content be aligned with IVDR!]

[129] Also called **Research Use Only products (RUOs)**; See MEDDEV 2.14/2 rev 1: IVD GUIDANCE: Research Use Only products; A GUIDE FOR MANUFACTURERS AND NOTIFIED BODIES [still to be adjusted to IVDR!]; do not confound these products with devices for performance studies!

[130] see also MEDDEV 2.14/1 rev 2 chapter 2.3. for examples under the IVDD [alignment with IVDR still necessary!]

Chapter 3: General Obligations of Economic Operators: Manufacturers, System&Procedure Pack Producers, Authorised Representatives, Importers, Distributors; Person Responsible for Regulatory Compliance (PRRC)

In the two regulations, the EU legislator - in accordance with the New Legal Framework - has for the first time explicitly summarised general obligations of the above-mentioned economic operators in the field of medical devices and IVDs:

3.1. Manufacturer

Art. 10 of both regulations lists the general obligations of the manufacturers, which are aimed to assure compliance with the requirements of the respective regulation over the entire life cycle of the products. In many respects, this must be accomplished under an **obligatory QMS**, which must ensure the conformity of the products and procedures throughout the life cycle of MDs/IVDs concerned.

'manufacturer' means a natural or legal person who manufactures or fully refurbishes a device or has a device designed, manufactured or fully refurbished, and markets that device under its name or trade mark;

General requirements of the obligatory QMS:
- Manufacturers of devices[131] shall establish, document, implement, maintain, keep up to date and continually improve a **quality management system (QMS)** that shall ensure compliance with this Regulation in the most effective manner and in a manner that is proportionate to the risk class and the type of device;
- The quality management system shall cover all parts and elements of a manufacturer's organisation dealing with the quality of processes, pro-

---

[131] MDR: other than investigational devices; IVDR: other than devices for performance studies

92

cedures and devices. It shall govern the structure, responsibilities, procedures, processes and management resources required to implement the principles and actions necessary to achieve compliance with the provisions of MDR/IVDR;

- Manufacturers shall ensure that procedures are in place to keep series production in conformity with the requirements of MDR/IVDR. Changes in device design or characteristics and changes in the harmonised standards or CS by reference to which the conformity of a device is declared shall be adequately taken into account in a timely manner;
- resource management, including selection and control of suppliers and sub-contractors;
- product realisation, including planning, design, development, production and service provision;
- processes for monitoring and measurement of output, data analysis and product improvement.

In addition to these general requirements of a QMS, **specific aspects of the QMS** have now to be explicitly targeted to specific aspects of the MD/IVD regulatory system. This applies in particular to:

- the **targeted management of regulatory compliance**[132] (screening and determination of the full regulatory profile MDs/IVDs must fulfill, including qualification, screening for other EU/nat. legislation applicable; classification; selection and handling of appropriate conformity assessment procedures; management of changes; identification of applicable general safety and performance requirements of Annex I and search for suitable solutions (in particular by means of harmonised European standards or CS or alternative solutions with justification) and
- **important life-cycle processes**[133], such as **risk management, clinical evaluation of MD (incl. PMCF), performance evaluation of IVD (incl. PMPF), post-market surveillance (PMS)** and **vigilance** [including report-

---

[132] See chapters 1.5, 2 and 11; 12 and 13; and chapter 5 of this book
[133] See chapters 5.1, 6, 7, 15 and 16 of this book

ing procedures and corrective and preventive actions (CAPA), and if necessary, Field Safety Corrective Actions (FSCA)]; **registration obligations in EUDAMED and UDI**[134], each process with the appropriate organisational structures, records, reports, procedures, methods, resources, competence, documentation and controls.

- The manufacturer must register as an economic operator (actor) in EUDAMED and receives a unique registration number (Single Registration Number - SRN).

See as currently (March 2022) harmonised standard for a QMS for regulatory purposes:
Medical devices - Quality management systems - Requirements for regulatory purposes (ISO 13485:2016) OJ L 1 - 05/01/2022[135]

The manufacturer must also fulfil the following obligations:
- ○ Execution of the **appropriate conformity assessment**, if necessary with change management[136] and consultation procedures[137];
- ○ Issue of the **EU Declaration of Conformity**[138],
- ○ Affixing the **CE marking**[139],
- ○ Preparation and updating of the **technical documentation** in accordance with Annex II and III of both Regulations,
- ○ Management of a **Post-Market Surveillance (PMS) System**[140],
- ○ Management of a **vigilance system**[141],
- ○ **Cooperation with stakeholders**, esp. the responsible competent authorities (CAs), including provision of relevant documents for proof

---

[134] See Chapter III and Annex VI in both Regulations; see chap. 4 in this book;

[135] See: https://ec.europa.eu/docsroom/documents/48579

[136] See esp. Annexes IX to XI in both Regulations; chap. 12 and 13 in this book;

[137] See chapter 12 and 13

[138] MDR: Art. 19 and Annex IV; IVDR: Art. 17 and Annex IV; consider national language requirements where marketing is planned within EU/EEA!

[139] MDR: Art. 20 and Annex V; IVDR: Art. 18 and Annex V

[140] MDR: Chapter VII.1; Art. 83 and Annex III; IVDR: Chapter VII.1; Art. 78 and Annex III; both: see chap. 15 in this book;

[141] Manufacturers shall have a system for recording and reporting of incidents and field safety corrective actions as described in Chapter VII.2. of both Regulations

of conformity and, if necessary, provision of samples or access to device on request; in the event of inadequate cooperation with the CA, significant sanctions are possible; the documents may also be made available by the CA to parties with legitimate interests in the event of justified suspicion of damage by an MD/IVD;

o   Natural and legal persons may claim damages in accordance with EU and national law in the event of damage caused by defective MDs/IVDs; manufacturers must ensure **sufficient financial cover for their potential liability** in accordance with the Product Liability Directive or any stricter national legislation.

o   For a manufacturer with a registered place of business outside the EU/EEA, the manufacturer must appoint one or more **authorised representatives** by mandate as defined in Art. 11 and 12;

o   Manufacturers shall ensure that the device is accompanied by the **information** set out in Annex I[142] in (an) official Union language(s) determined by the Member State(s) in which the device is made available to the user or patient. The particulars on the label shall be indelible, easily legible and clearly comprehensible to the intended user or patient.

o   Manufacturers who consider or have reason to believe that a device which they have placed on the market or put into service is not in conformity with this Regulation shall immediately take the necessary corrective action to bring that device into conformity, to withdraw it or to recall it, as appropriate. They shall inform the distributors of the device in question and, where applicable, the authorised representative and importers accordingly. Where the device presents a serious risk, manufacturers shall immediately inform the competent authorities of the Member States in which they made the device available and, where applicable, the notified body that issued a certificate for the device in accordance with MDR: Article 56; IVDR: Art. 51, in particular, of the non-compliance and of any corrective action taken.

---

[142] MDR: Annex I, Section 23; IVDR: Section 20 of Annex I

3.2. System&Procedure Pack[143] Producer (SPPP)

MDR: Art. 22

Guidance: MDCG 2018-4: Definitions/descriptions and formats of the UDI core elements for systems or procedure packs

MDCG 2018-3 Rev1: Guidance on UDI for systems and procedure packs (SPPP receive in EUDAMED an Actor-ID, which is not an SRN!);

MDCG 2021-13Rev1: Questions and answers on obligations and related rules for the registration in EUDAMED of actors other than manufacturers, authorised representatives and importers subject to the obligations of Article 31 MDR and Article 28 IVDR (*important for EUDAMED registration for EU- and non EU-based SPPP!; see specifically chapter 6 und 7 of this MDCG 2021-13Rev1*)

These natural or legal persons (organisations) put together CE-marked MDs with other CE-marked MDs or IVDs[144] and/or other products in accordance with the intended purpose/use given by their respective manufacturers in order to place them on the market as a system or procedure pack. These other products have to be in conformity with legislation that applies to those products and they are to be used within a medical procedure or their presence in the system or procedure pack is otherwise medically justified.

- o The producer has to issue a statement acc. to MDR: Art. 22 (2)[145];
- o The systems or procedure packs shall not themselves bear an additional CE marking but the labelling shall clearly identify the producer and its location, where it can be contacted;
- o the information acc. to MDR: Annex I.23 of the combined products have to accompany the combination;

---

[143] MDR: Art. 2 (10) *'procedure pack' means a combination of products packaged together and placed on the market with the purpose of being used for a specific medical purpose;*
(11) 'system' means a combination of products, either packaged together or not, which are intended to be inter-connected or combined to achieve a specific medical purpose;
[144] CE-marked under the IVDR
[145] To be kept at the disposal of the competent authorities for ≥ 10/15 years acc to MDR: Art. 10 (8)

- for registration in EUDAMED see the above mentioned MDCG guidances;
- there are specific provisions in MDR: Art. 22 (3) for any natural or legal person who sterilises systems or procedure packs for the purpose of placing them on the market. These persons shall at their choice, apply one of the conformity assessment procedures set out in MDR: Annex IX or the procedure set out in Part A of Annex XI limited to the aspects of sterility. The natural or legal person shall draw up a statement declaring that sterilisation has been carried out in accordance with the manufacturers instructions.
- Where the system or procedure pack incorporates devices which do not bear the CE marking or where the chosen combination of devices is not compatible in view of their original intended purpose, or where the sterilisation has not been carried out in accordance with the manufacturer's instructions, the system or procedure pack shall be treated as a device in its own right and shall be subject to the relevant conformity assessment procedure pursuant to MDR: Article 52. The natural or legal person shall assume the obligations incumbent on manufacturers.

3.3. Authorized Representative

Articles 11 and 12 of both Regulations
Factsheet for Authorised Representatives, Importers and Distributors of medical devices and in vitro diagnostic medical devices[146]

> *'authorised representative'* means any natural or legal person established within the Union who has received and accepted a written mandate from a manufacturer, located outside the Union, to act on the manufacturer's behalf in relation to specified tasks with regard to the latter's obligations under this Regulation;

Every manufacturer outside the EU/EEA needs an authorized representative as direct contact person for the competent authorities in the EU/EEA for the

---

[146] https://ec.europa.eu/health/medical-devices-new-regulations/getting-ready-new-regulations/authorised-representatives-importers-and-distributors_en

placing on the market or putting into service of an MD/IVD. This authorised representative has to be designated by the manufacturer by <u>mandate</u> exclusively for one, several or all of his generic product groups. This mandate must contain defined generic product groups and assigned tasks, may not contain certain tasks defined in Art. 11 (4) and must be accepted in writing by the authorised representative. If the manufacturer acts contrary to his obligations under the Regulation, the authorized representative shall terminate the contract and inform his competent authority and, if applicable, the NB accordingly.

The authorised representative has to perform the following tasks:

(a) verify that the EU declaration of conformity and technical documentation have been drawn up and, where applicable, that an appropriate conformity assessment procedure has been carried out by the manufacturer;

(b) keep available a copy of the technical documentation, the EU declaration of conformity and, if applicable, a copy of the relevant certificate, including any amendments and supplements, issued in accordance with MDR: Art. 56/IVDR: Art. 51, at the disposal of competent authorities for the period referred to in Article 10(8)[147];

(c) comply with the registration obligations laid down in Article 31 and verify that the manufacturer has complied with the registration obligations laid down in Articles 27 and 29;

(d) in response to a request from a competent authority, provide that competent authority with all the information and documentation necessary to demonstrate the conformity of a device, in an official Union language determined by the Member State concerned;

(e) forward to the manufacturer any request by a competent authority of the Member State in which the authorised representative has its registered place of business for samples, or access to a device and verify that the competent authority receives the samples or is given access to the device;

(f) cooperate with the competent authorities on any preventive or corrective action taken to eliminate or, if that is not possible, mitigate the risks posed by devices;

---

[147] To be kept at the disposal of the competent authorities for ≥ 10/(15 for implants) years acc to MDR: Art. 10 (8); ≥ 10y acc. to IVDR:Art. 10 (7), after placing on the market of the last product

(g) immediately inform the manufacturer about complaints and reports from healthcare professionals, patients and users about suspected incidents related to a device for which they have been designated;
(h) terminate the mandate if the manufacturer acts contrary to its obligations under this Regulation.

The mandate referred to in paragraph 3 of this Article shall not delegate the manufacturer's obligations laid down in Article 10(1), (2), (3), (4), (6), (7), (9), (10), (11) and (12).

Without prejudice to paragraph 4 of Art. 11, where the manufacturer is not established in a Member State and has not complied with the obligations laid down in Article 10, the authorised representative shall be legally liable for defective devices on the same basis as, and jointly and severally with, the manufacturer.

An authorised representative who terminates its mandate on the ground referred to in point (h) of paragraph 3 shall immediately inform the competent authority of the Member State in which it is established and, where applicable, the notified body that was involved in the conformity assessment for the device of the termination of the mandate and the reasons therefor.

Any reference in MDR/IVDR to the competent authority of the Member State in which the manufacturer has its registered place of business shall be understood as a reference to the competent authority of the Member State in which the authorised representative, designated by a manufacturer has its registered place of business.
If the manufacturer does not fulfil his obligations under Art. 10, the authorised representative is jointly and severally liable for defective products on the same basis as the manufacturer!

The authorised representative receives a unique registration number (Single Registration Number - SRN) in EUDAMED.

Art. 12 deals with the change of an authorised representative and the modalities for a proper transfer/acceptance of obligations.

3.4. Importer

Art. 13 of both Regulations
MDCG 2021-27: Questions and Answers on Articles 13 & 14 of Regulation (EU) 2017/745 and Regulation (EU) 2017/746
Factsheet for Authorised Representatives, Importers and Distributors of medical devices and in vitro diagnostic medical devices[148]

> *'importer'[149] means any natural or legal person established within the Union that places a device from a third country on the Union market;*

Importers may only place MDs/IVDs on the market that comply with MDR/IVDR. To this end, it has various verification obligations:

- the device has been CE marked and that the EU declaration of conformity of the device has been drawn up;
- a manufacturer is identified and that an authorised representative in accordance with Article 11 has been designated by the manufacturer; this would include verification, that both have also fulfilled their registration obligations in EUDAMED[150];
- the device is labelled in accordance with this Regulation and accompanied by the required instructions for use;
- where applicable, a UDI has been assigned by the manufacturer in accordance with Article 27 of MDR resp. Art. 24 of IVDR;
- the device is registered in EUDAMED; importers will add their details to the registration[151];
- the importer has to keep a copy of the EU Declaration of conformity and of any relevant (NB) certificate, incl. any amendments or supplements for the period given in Art. 10 (8) of MDR and Art. 10 (7) of IVDR[152].

The importer must make himself "visible":

1) on the product, its labelling or on a document accompanying the device:

---

[148] https://ec.europa.eu/health/medical-devices-new-regulations/getting-ready-new-regulations/authorised-representatives-importers-and-distributors_en
[149] MDR: Art. 2 (33)/IVDR: Art 2 (26)
[150] See MDR: Art. 30 (3); IVDR: Art. 27 (3)
[151] MDR: Art. 31; IVDR: Art. ; see also Annex VI, Part A.1 of MDR/IVDR
[152] 10 years after the last product has been placed on the market; 15 years for implantables

- Importers name, registered trade name or registered trade mark;
- registered place of business and the address at which they can be contacted, so that their location can be established;

2) they have to register in EUDAMED as an economic operator (actor)[153] and receive a Single Registration Number – SRN; they have to add their details to the product registration[154];

The importer has to cooperate as concerns Post Market Surveillance, vigilance and market surveillance with other economic operators (manufacturer [MF]; authorised representative [AR]; distributors [DIST]) and competent authorities (CA), also as a result of it's verification tasks, as indicated above:

- Where an importer considers or has reason to believe that a device is not in conformity with the requirements of the relevant Regulation, it shall not place the device on the market until it has been brought into conformity and shall inform the manufacturer and the manufacturer's authorised representative; Importers shall keep a register of complaints, of non-conforming devices and of recalls and withdrawals, and provide the MF, AR and DIST with any information requested by them, in order to allow them to investigate complaints.

- Importers who consider or have reason to believe that a device which they have placed on the market is not in conformity with this Regulation shall immediately inform the MF and its AR. Importers shall co-operate with the MF, the MF's AR and the CA's to ensure that the necessary corrective action to bring that device into conformity, to withdraw or recall it is taken. Where the device presents a serious risk, they shall also immediately inform the CAs of the Member States in which they made the device available and, if applicable, the notified body that issued a certificate in accordance with MDR: Art. 56/IVDR: Art. 52 for the device in question, giving details, in particular, of the non-compliance and of any corrective action taken;

---

[153] MDR: Art. 31; IVDR: Art. 28
[154] see Annex VI, Part A.1 of MDR/IVDR

- Importers have to fulfil their <u>traceability requirements</u> (up- and down-stream) acc. to MDR: Art. 25 resp. IVDR: Art. 22;
- Importers who have received complaints or reports from healthcare professionals, patients or users about suspected incidents related to a device which they have placed on the market shall immediately forward this information to the MF and its AR;
- Importers shall cooperate with CAs, at the latters' request, on any action taken to eliminate or, if that is not possible, mitigate the risks posed by devices which they have placed on the market. Importers, upon request by a CA of the Member State in which the importer has its registered place of business, shall provide samples of the device free of charge or, where that is impracticable, grant access to the device.

Importers have to assure correct storage and transport conditions:
- Importers shall ensure that, while a device is under their responsibility, storage or transport conditions do not jeopardise its compliance with the general safety and performance requirements set out in Annex I and shall comply with the conditions set by the MF, where available.

3.5. Distributor

Art. 14 of both Regulations
MDCG 2021-27: Questions and Answers on Articles 13 & 14 of Regulation (EU) 2017/745 and Regulation (EU) 2017/746
Factsheet for Authorised Representatives, Importers and Distributors of medical devices and in vitro diagnostic medical devices[155].

> *'distributor'[156] means any natural or legal person in the supply chain, other than the manufacturer or the importer, that makes a device available on the market, up until the point of putting into service;*

---

[155] https://ec.europa.eu/health/medical-devices-new-regulations/getting-ready-new-regulations/authorised-representatives-importers-and-distributors_en
[156] MDR: Art. 2 (34) and IVDR: Art. 2 (27)

Before placing products on the market, the distributor has some obligations to verify, that the product is in conformity with the relevant regulation: This verification exercise would include the following feasibility checks (partly on a representative basis):

- Is the product CE marked and has a Declaration of conformity been issued?
- Is the device is accompanied by the information to be supplied by the manufacturer in accordance with MDR: Art. 10(11); IVDR: Art. 10 (10)[157];
- for imported devices, the importer has complied with the requirements set out in Article 13(3)[158];
- that, where applicable, a UDI has been assigned by the manufacturer.

The 1st, 2nd and 4th point may be checked at a representative basis.

The **distributor has to cooperate as concerns Post Market Surveillance, vigilance and market surveillance** with other economic operators (manufacturer [MF]; authorised representative [AR]; distributors [DIST]) and with competent authorities (CA), also as a result of its verification tasks, as indicated above:

- Where a distributor considers or has reason to believe that a <u>device is not in conformity</u> with the requirements of this Regulation, it shall not make the device available on the market until it has been brought into conformity, and shall inform the manufacturer and, where applicable, the manufacturer's authorised representative, and the importer. Where the distributor considers or has reason to believe that the device presents a <u>serious risk or is a falsified device</u>, it shall also inform the competent authority of the Member State in which it is established.
- Distributors that consider or have reason to believe that a device which they have made available on the market is <u>not in conformity</u> with this Regulation shall immediately inform the manufacturer and, where applicable, the manufacturer's authorised representative and the importer. Distributors shall co-operate with the manufacturer and, where

---

[157] Information acc. to Annex I.III.23 of MDR or Annex I.III.20 of IVDR in the appropriate language(s)

[158] See "visibility" requirements of importer, as above

applicable, the manufacturer's authorised representative, and the importer, and with competent authorities to ensure that the <u>necessary corrective action to bring that device into conformity, to withdraw or to recall</u> it, as appropriate, is taken. Where the distributor considers or has reason to believe that the <u>device presents a serious risk</u>, it shall also immediately inform the competent authorities of the Member States in which it made the device available, giving details, in particular, of the non-compliance and of any corrective action taken.

- Distributors have to fulfil their <u>traceability requirements</u> (up- and downstream) acc. to MDR: Art. 25 resp. IVDR: Art. 22;
- Distributors that have <u>received complaints or reports from healthcare professionals, patients or users about suspected incidents</u> related to a device they have made available, shall immediately forward this information to the manufacturer and, where applicable, the manufacturer's authorised representative, and the importer. They shall keep a <u>register of complaints, of non-conforming devices and of recalls and withdrawals</u>, and keep the manufacturer and, where available, the authorised representative and the importer informed of such monitoring and provide them with any information upon their request.
- Distributors shall, upon request by a competent authority, provide it with all the information and documentation that is at their disposal and is necessary to demonstrate the conformity of a device.

Distributors shall be considered to have fulfilled the obligation referred to in the above subparagraph when the manufacturer or, where applicable, the authorised representative for the device in question provides the required information.

- Distributors shall cooperate with competent authorities, at their request, on any action taken to eliminate the risks posed by devices which they have made available on the market. Distributors, upon request by a competent authority, shall provide free samples of the device or, where that is impracticable, grant access to the device.

Distributors have to assure correct storage and transport conditions:

- Distributors shall ensure that, while a device is under their responsibility, storage or transport conditions do not jeopardise its compliance with the general safety and performance requirements set out in Annex I and shall comply with the conditions set by the Manufacturer, where available.

3.6. Person Responsible for Regulatory Compliance (PRRC)

Art. 15 of both Regulations
MDCG 2019-7: Guidance on article 15 of the medical device regulation (MDR) and in vitro diagnostic device regulation (IVDR) on a 'person responsible for regulatory compliance' (PRRC)[159]

By analogy to the "Qualified Person" in the pharmaceutical sector and the "safety officers" already established in several national Medical Device Laws, for example in AT, FR and DE, the MDR/IVDR now establishes one (or more) person(s) for compliance with the regulatory requirements that the manufacturer must have in his organisation. Micro and small enterprises[160] and authorised representatives do not need to have this person available in their organisation, but must have permanently and continuously such a person at their disposal.

The required **specialist knowledge** of this person in the MD/IVD area must be proven
  a) by a **relevant university degree** and at least **one year of professional experience in regulatory affairs or QMS** in conjunction with MD/IVD[161].

---

[159] https://ec.europa.eu/health/md_sector/new_regulations/guidance_en
[160] See Commission Recommendation of 6 May 2003 concerning the definition of micro, small and medium-sized enterprises (OJ L 124, 20.5.2003, p. 36):
micro enterprise: fewer than 10 employees and an annual turnover (the amount of money taken in a particular period) or balance sheet (a statement of a company's assets and liabilities) below €2 million.
small enterprise: fewer than 50 employees and an annual turnover or balance sheet below €10 million.
medium-sized enterprise: fewer than 250 employees and annual turnover below €50 million or balance sheet below €43 million.
[161] Please note that in both Regulations this experience is formally not transferred to the other sector (MD<≠>IVD)

b) Alternatively, **4 years of professional experience in regulatory affairs or QMS** in connection with MD/IVD are sufficient.

Manufacturers of **custom-made devices** can prove the required specialist knowledge by **2 years of professional experience in a corresponding manufacturing area** (depending on national regulations).

Tab. 6 MDR/IVDR: Minimum Responsibilities of the PRRC

The **task profile/responsibility of the PRRC includes** that he ensures:
o the product is released only after checking appropriately the conformity of products within the framework of the QMS for production,   o the technical documentation and EU declaration of conformity are drawn up and kept up to date,   o the obligations arising from the PMS and the reporting obligations under the vigilance system are fulfilled,   o the Statement on the general safety and performance requirements for investigational devices (MD)/devices for performance studies (IVD) has been issued.

Chapter 4. European Databank EUDAMED and its Modules; UDI-System; Identification and Traceability of MD/IVD; European Medical Device Nomenclature (EMDN)

Legal Sources:

Chapter III and Annex VI of both Regulations

Non-legally binding Guidance:

MDCG endorsed documents[162]:

UDI:

MDCG 2021-19: Guidance note integration of the UDI within an organisation's quality management system

MDCG 2021-10: The status of Appendixes E-I of IMDRF N48 under the EU regulatory framework for medical devices

MDCG 2021-09: MDCG Position Paper on the Implementation of UDI requirements for contact lenses, spectacle frames, spectacle lenses & ready readers

MDCG 2020-18: MDCG Position Paper on UDI assignment for Spectacle lenses & Ready readers

MDCG 2019-2: Guidance on application of UDI rules to device-part of products referred to in article 1(8), 1(9) and 1(10) of Regulation 745/2017

MDCG 2019-1: MDCG guiding principles for issuing entities rules on basic UDI-DI

MDCG 2018-7: Provisional considerations regarding language issues associated with the UDI database

MDCG 2018-6: Clarifications of UDI related responsibilities in relation to article 16

MDCG 2018-5: UDI assignment to medical device software

MDCG 2018-4: Definitions/descriptions and formats of the UDI core elements for systems or procedure packs

MDCG 2018-3 Rev.1: Guidance on UDI for systems and procedure packs

---

[162] See here all present and forthcoming MDCG Guidances: http://ec.europa.eu/growth/sectors/medical-devices/guidance_en

MDCG 2018-2: Future EU medical device nomenclature - Description of requirements

MDCG 2018-1 v3: Guidance on basic UDI-DI and changes to UDI-DI

EUDAMED[163]:

MDCG 2021-13 rev.1: Questions and answers on obligations and related
rules for the registration in EUDAMED of actors other than manufacturers, authorised representatives and importers subject to the obligations
of Article 31 MDR and Article 28 IVDR

MDCG 2021-1 rev.1: Guidance on harmonised administrative practices and
alternative technical solutions until EUDAMED is fully functional

MDCG 2020-15: MDCG Position Paper on the use of the EUDAMED actor
registration module and of the Single Registration Number (SRN) in the
Member States

MDCG 2019-5: Registration of legacy devices in EUDAMED

MDCG 2019-4: Timelines for registration of device data elements in EU-
DAMED

European Medical Device Nomenclature (EMDN)[164]

MDCG 2021-12: FAQ on the European Medical Device Nomenclature
(EMDN)

The EMDN – The nomenclature of use in EUDAMED

The CND nomenclature – Background and general principles

GHTF/IMDRF Guidance: (non-legally binding)

UDI Guidance: Unique Device Identification (UDI) of Medical Devices[165]

---

[163] For a survey and state of play: https://ec.europa.eu/health/medical-devices-eu-
damed/overview_en

[164] https://ec.europa.eu/health/medical-devices-sector/new-regulations/guidance-mdcg-
endorsed-documents-and-other-guidance_en#sec5

[165] http://www.imdrf.org/docs/imdrf/final/technical/imdrf-tech-131209-udi-guidance-
140901.pdf#search=%22udi%22

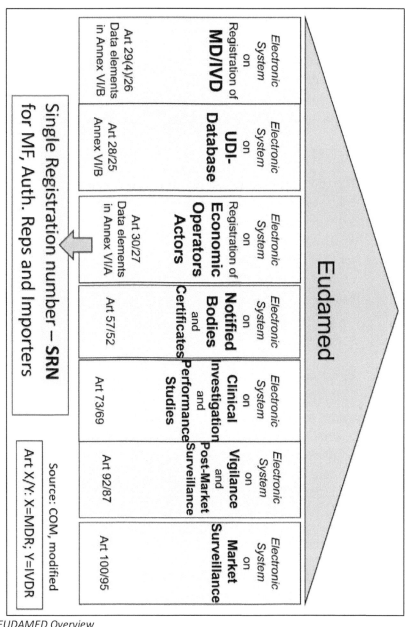

Fig. 12 EUDAMED Overview

4.1. European Database EUDAMED

The transparency and functionality of the MD/IVD regulatory system for all stakeholders and the public is to be ensured in future by a powerful European database: EUDAMED.

EUDAMED[166] contains the following interconnected modules (electronic systems - ES; see Fig. 12) **EUDAMED restricted** and a public website: **EUDAMED public.**

The modules of EUDAMED:

- The ES for the **registration of economic operators**[167] (manufacturers, authorised representatives, importers, to each of which a unique registration number (Single Registration Number - SRN) is assigned; system&procedure pack producers (SPPP) will have an Actor ID which is not an SRN[168];
- ES for the **registration of MD/IVD** in connection with the **UDI-database**;
- ES for **Notified Bodies (NB) and their certificates**;
- ES for **clinical investigations** of MD and for **performance studies** of IVD;
- ES for **vigilance** and **post-market surveillance (PMS)**;
- ES for **market surveillance**;

The provisions on the new EUDAMED[169] database in principle will not enter into force until an independent audit has shown its functionality and the COM has published a communication to that effect in the Official Journal. As the regular date for the communication (25 March 2021) has been missed by the COM, EUDAMED (the modules for actors, Vigilance, Clinical Investiga-

---

[166] https://ec.europa.eu/health/md_eudamed/overview_en

[167] https://ec.europa.eu/health/sites/health/files/md_sector/docs/2020-15-position-paper-actor-registration-module_en.pdf

[168] See also: MDCG 2021-13 Rev.1: Questions and answers on obligations and related rules for the registration in EUDAMED of actors other than manufacturers, authorised representatives and importers subject to the obligations of Article 31 MDR and Article 28 IVDR

[169] For a survey and state of play of EUDAMED, see: https://ec.europa.eu/health/medical-devices-eudamed/overview_en

tion&Performance Studies, and Market surveillance)) would become mandatory 6 months after such a delayed communication by the COM. Product/UDI module and NB&Certificate registration become mandatory 24 months after the COM Publication in the OJEU. (see MDR: Art. 123 (d) and (e)). Details on the current time-frames, see chapter I.6 in this book.

The Commission Implementing Regulation (EU) 2021/2078 of 26 November 2021 lays down the detailed arrangements necessary for the setting up and maintenance of EUDAMED.

The Commission, in agreement with the Medical Device Coordination Group (MDCG), is currently going to make available the different modules on a gradual and voluntary basis as soon as they are functional:

The module on Actor registration for MDR is available voluntarily since December 2020; the module on UDI and product registration and the module on Certificates and Notified Bodies since October 2021. Afterwards, the remaining modules will be made available voluntarily, as soon as they are functional.

When an economic operator has submitted its actor registration request, the selected relevant national competent authority issues the SRN (generated by EUDAMED) after approving the registration request. EUDAMED notifies the SRN via email to the economic operator.

Access to MDR EUDAMED restricted is restricted to users identified by their EU Login account. To create your account please go to: https://webgate.ec.europa.eu/cas/login .

Actor registration:

For an overview of the actor registration request process please see:
https://ec.europa.eu/health/medical-devices-eudamed/actor-registration-module_en#user-guide-for-economic-operators and here:
https://ec.europa.eu/health/sites/health/files/md_eudamed/docs/md_actor_registration_request_process_en.pdf

For a more detailed instruction of actor registration you may look here:

Guide to Using EUDAMED - Actor registration module for economic operators[170] and MDCG 2021-13 Rev.1 (for actors that would only receive an Actor-ID, which is not an SRN)[171]

UDI/devices registration:
A comprehensive overview is presented by the COM here:
https://ec.europa.eu/health/medical-devices-eudamed/udidevices-registration_en
A more detailed guide is given here:
UDI/DEVICES USER GUIDE
https://ec.europa.eu/health/document/download/bf8d449d-e2a2-4cb2-bee3-bace11f58b5e_en
Notified Bodies and Certificates module:
The COM provides comprehensive information on this module here:
https://ec.europa.eu/health/medical-devices-eudamed/notified-bodies-and-certificates-module_en

EUDAMED public may be searched here (currently for the 3 modules, which have been made available voluntarily):
https://ec.europa.eu/tools/eudamed/#/screen/home

4.2. UDI-System[172]

MDR: Art. 27 and 28; IVDR: Art. 24 and 25; Annex VI of both Regulations.
MDCG Guidances: see here[173]

---

[170] https://ec.europa.eu/health/medical-devices-eudamed/actor-registration-module_en#user-guide-for-economic-operators
[171] MDCG 2021-13Rev.1: Questions and answers on obligations and related rules for the registration in EUDAMED of actors other than manufacturers, authorised representatives and importers subject to the obligations of Article 31 MDR and Article 28 IVDR
[172] https://ec.europa.eu/health/md_topics-interest/unique_device_identifier_en
[173] https://ec.europa.eu/health/medical-devices-sector/new-regulations/guidance-mdcg-endorsed-documents-and-other-guidance_en#sec12

Medtech Europe: MedTech Europe guidance for assigning Basic UDI-DI[174]

On the basis of preliminary work on a global level (GHTF/IMDRF), both Regulations adopt the **UDI system for clear product identification and support of traceability** in the medical devices/IVD area[175].

The unique device identification (UDI) is a unique numeric or alphanumeric code related to a medical device/IVD. It allows for a clear and unambiguous identification of specific devices on the market and facilitates their traceability. The UDI codes comprise the following components

- a device identifier (UDI-DI)
- a Basic UDI-DI, and
- a production identifier (UDI-PI)

These provide rapid access to useful and specific information about the device. The specificity of the UDI

- makes traceability of devices more efficient
- allows easier recall or withdrawal of devices
- helps combat counterfeiting
- improves patient safety
- serves public health

The UDI will supplement (not replace!) the existing labelling requirements for medical devices in the EU.

This UDI system consists of the following elements:
o The **production of a UDI** by the manufacturer in accordance with a UDI issuing entity (see below), which he allocates to the product and, if applicable, to all higher packaging levels[176], consisting of:
o A **UDI Device identifier (UDI-DI)** specific to the manufacturer, the MD/IVD and its packaging level;

---

[174] https://www.medtecheurope.org/wp-content/uploads/2020/06/200602_MTE-Basic-UDI-DI-guidance-v1.1_final.pdf
[175] Except custom made MD and investigational devices and devices for performance studies
[176] A shipping container is not considered a higher level of packaging for UDI

- o A **Basic UDI DI** as an identifier of the product model[177]; it is the DI assigned at the level of the device unit of use; and
- o A **UDI production identifier (UDI-PI)**[178]

- o Placing of the UDI on the product label or on its packaging using the **UDI carrier**, which may be human-readable (human readable information; HRI) and/or machine-readable (Automatic Identification and Data Capture; AIDC), like bar codes, data matrix codes or RFID;
- o The **storage of the UDI** by economic actors, health institutions and health care professionals within the framework of the traceability of certain products;
- o An electronic system for unique product identification (**UDI database**) in which essential product data (acc. to Annex VI.B of both regulations) is uploaded and stored;
- o Appropriate **UDI issuing entities** that operate a UDI assignment system reliably for at least 5[179] years and are designated by the COM[180].

---

4 UDI issuing entities have been designated by the COM:
- (a) GS1 AISBL
- (b) Health Industry Business Communications Council (HIBCC)
- (c) ICCBBA
- (d) Informationsstelle für Arzneispezialitäten — IFA GmbH

The UDI system, in particular the attachment of the UDI carriers to the product will come into force in stages according to the risk classes of the products (see section I.6. in this book).

---

[177] The Basic UDI-DI is the primary identifier of a device model. It is the DI assigned at the level of the device unit of use. It is the main key for records in the UDI database and is referenced in relevant NB-certificates and EU Declarations of Conformity. For details see MDCG 2018-1v3 and MDCG 2019-1

[178] The UDI-PI is a numeric or alphanumeric code that identifies the unit of device production. The different types of UDI-PI(s) include serial number, lot number, software identification and manufacturing or expiry date or both types of date.

[179] Initially in the regulations at least 10 years envisaged

[180] COMMISSION IMPLEMENTING DECISION (EU) 2019/939 of 6 June 2019 designating issuing entities designated to operate a system for the assignment of Unique Device Identifiers (UDIs) in the field of medical devices

4.3. Traceability (Identification within the supply chain)[181]

All economic operators in the supply chain shall co-operate to achieve an appropriate level of traceability of devices. This is particularly important for the Post-Market Surveillance System and the Vigilance system (see chapters XV and XVI of this book)

Economic operators shall be able to identify the following to the competent authority, for a period of at least 10 years[182] (implantable MDs for a period of at least 15 years)[183]:

(a) any economic operator to whom they have directly supplied a device;

(b) any economic operator who has directly supplied them with a device;

(c) any health institution or healthcare professional to which they have directly supplied a device.

Economic operators must store and keep (preferably by electronic means) the UDI of devices they have supplied or have been supplied with for **class III implantable MDs** and for MDs or IVDs for which the COM has introduced such an obligation by implementing act.

Health institutions must store and keep (preferably by electronic means) the UDI of devices they have supplied or have been supplied with for **class III implantable MDs.**

Member States must encourage, and may require, health institutions and health care professionals to store and keep, preferably by electronic means, the UDI of the devices with which they have been supplied.

4.4. European Medical Device Nomenclature (EMDN)

MDR: Art. 26 and IVDR Art. 23 oblige the COM in connection with EU-DAMED to provide an internationally applicable nomenclature for medical devices to economic operators and other stakeholders (including healthcare

---

[181] MDR: Art. 25 and Art. 27 (8), (9) and (11); IVDR: Art. 22 and Art. 24 (8) and (11)

[182] After the last device covered by the EU Declaration of Conformity has been placed on the market

[183] MDR: Art. 25; IVDR: Art. 22: after placing the last product on the market

facilities) as free of charge as possible[184]. The European Medical Device Nomenclature (EMDN) will be the nomenclature used by manufacturers when registering their medical devices in the database EUDAMED. On the basis of predefined criteria and requirements from MDCG 2018-2: "Future EU medical Device nomenclature, Description of requirements" and on the basis of guidelines from the Medical Device Coordination Group (MDCG), the European Commission has opted for the use of the "Classificazione Nazionale Dispositivi medici (CND)" as the basis for the EMDN. An extraordinary revision of the CND has paved the way to release the first version of the EMDN, that will be integrated into EUDAMED for use by the actors. The EMDN will be fully available and accessible to all operators and will be free of copyright. As far as possible, the Commission will map the EMDN to the Global Medical Device Nomenclature (GMDN). This task has been undertaken in the hope, that the search for EMDN codes by operators currently using GMDN may be facilitated. The correspondences between the nomenclatures will be visible to the operators and will be included in the future database in the form of a search tool. For this reason, and in collaboration with GMDN, the mapping excercise is currently being carried out. The level of quality and reliability of this mapping exercise depends on the commitment of all relevant parties to cooperate in the mapping and validation of the results. A sub-group of the MDCG on nomenclature, which includes experts from the relevant national authorities and stakeholders has been established to oversee regulatory activities related to nomenclature.

In addition, the Commission is currently working with the World Health Organisation (WHO) on a future international nomenclature for medical devices.

The structure of EMDN:

The EMDN is characterised by its alphanumeric structure that is established in a seven-level hierarchical tree. It clusters medical devices into three main levels (see Fig. 13, out of MDCG 2021-12):

• Categories: the first hierarchical level,

• Groups: the second hierarchical level,

• Types: the third hierarchical level (which expands into several levels of detail (1°, 2°, 3°, 4° and 5°), where necessary.

---

[184] See https://webgate.ec.europa.eu/dyna2/emdn/ , where you can also download the most up to date version of the EMDN

Each alphanumeric code begins with a letter referring to the 'CATEGORY' to which the device falls under, followed by two numbers indicating the 'GROUP' and a series of numbers which refer to the 'TYPE'. The maximum number of digits is set at 13 (see Fig. 14, out of MDCG 2021-12).

Using the tree-like hierarchy of EMDN, users must always assign the most granular and terminal term available (lowest level in the tree) to their device.

Fig. 13 EMDN structure, from MDCG 2021-12

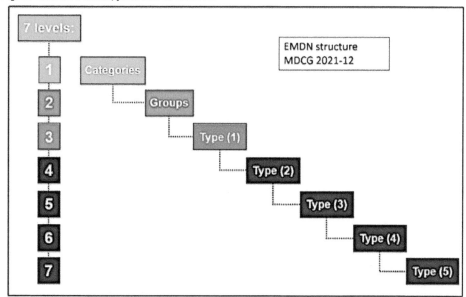

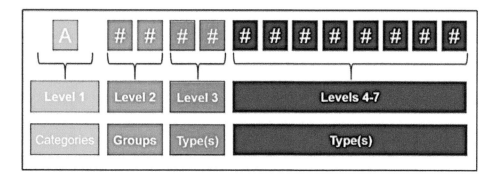

Fig. 14 EMDN alphanumeric code, from MDCG 2021-12

Chapter 5. General Safety and Performance Requirements for Medical Devices and IVDs

Annex I of both Regulations

Harmonized Standards with their Annexes Z and alternatives

According to the principles of the New Approach, the MDR/IVDR define in their Annex I the General Safety and Performance Requirements for MD and IVD (GSPR; see the survey in Figs. 17 and 18).

The previous corresponding term under the Directives has been: *Essential Requirements – ER*; in GHTF/IMDRF[185] and ISO[186] terminology they figure under *Essential Principles of Safety and Performance*).

Medical devices and IVDs must meet the applicable[187] General Safety and Performance Requirements.

Annex I contains 3 chapters:

Chapter I with the general requirements, which relate (very generally worded) to clinical evaluation of MDs in MDR[188] resp. performance evaluation of IVDs in IVDR[189] and (in a more specific way) to risk management

---

[185] www.imdrf.org

[186] ISO 16142-1:2016 Medical devices — Recognized essential principles of safety and performance of medical devices — Part 1: General essential principles and additional specific essential principles for all non-IVD medical devices and guidance on the selection of standards; ISO 16142-2:2017 Medical devices — Recognized essential principles of safety and performance of medical devices — Part 2: General essential principles and additional specific essential principles for all IVD medical devices and guidance on the selection of standards

[187] eg. Requirements for pharmaceutical components or for radiation protection will not be applicable to each and every MD/IVD

[188] See chapter VI in this book; MDR: Art. 5 (3): *3. Demonstration of conformity with the general safety and performance requirements shall include a clinical evaluation in accordance with Article 61.*
MDR: Art. 61 (1): *1. Confirmation of conformity with relevant general safety and performance requirements set out in Annex I under the normal conditions of the intended use of the device, and the evaluation of the undesirable side-effects and of the acceptability of the benefit-risk- ratio referred to in Sections 1 and 8 of Annex I, shall be based on clinical data providing sufficient clinical evidence, including where applicable relevant data as referred to in Annex III.*

[189] See chapter VII in this book; IVDR: Art. 5 (3): *3.Demonstration of conformity with the general safety and performance requirements shall include a performance evaluation in accordance with Article 56.*

(MDR/IVDR), based on a risk management plan for each MD/IVD, see below and Fig. 15.

Chapter II relates to (MDR): REQUIREMENTS REGARDING DESIGN AND MANUFACTURE and (in IVDR) to: REQUIREMENTS REGARDING PERFORMANCE[190], DESIGN AND MANUFACTURE.

These requirements will guide the necessary evaluation of the MD or IVD along the risk management during product design and realisation and will assist documentation necessary for the Technical Documentation acc. to Annex II and III.

Chapter III relates to REQUIREMENTS REGARDING INFORMATION SUPPLIED WITH THE DEVICE, esp. for labelling and instructions for use.

MDs/IVDs, which are also **machines** within the meaning of Directive 2006/42/EC, may also have to meet the essential health and safety requirements of Annex I to this Directive.

GSPR are specified by **harmonised European standards**, the references (titles) of which have been published in the Official Journal of the EU for this Regulation (formerly Directives)[191]. These standards each contain Annexes Z (ZA, ZB, …) which set out in detail which specific sections of the relevant standard provide a presumption of conformity to a certain GSPR (or a subitem of it) of the respective Regulation. Whereas harmonised European

---

IVDR: Art. 56 (1): *1.Confirmation of conformity with relevant general safety and performance requirements set out in Annex I, in particular those concerning the performance characteristics referred to in Chapter I and Section 9 of Annex I, under the normal conditions of the intended use of the device, and the evaluation of the interference(s) and cross-reaction(s) and of the acceptability of the benefit-risk ratio referred to in Sections 1 and 8 of Annex I, shall be based on scientific validity, analytical and clinical performance data providing sufficient clinical evidence, including where applicable relevant data as referred to in Annex III.*

[190] IVDR: Annex I.II.9. with performance requirements in fact belongs to the performance evaluation of IVDs

[191] for MDR, see: https://ec.europa.eu/growth/single-market/european-standards/harmonised-standards/medical-devices_en

for IVDR, see: https://ec.europa.eu/growth/single-market/european-standards/harmonised-standards/iv-diagnostic-medical-devices_en

standards grant conformity presumptions for certain aspects of the Regulation via these Annexes Z, they are not binding[192]. Instead, the manufacturer may also fulfil certain applicable GSPR or other requirements (like those e.g. for clinical investigations, performance studies, risk management or Post-market surveillance) of the Regulation by other means, with detailed reasoning and justification. These other means may often be, e.g. in the absence harmonised standards, available state of the art standards[193]. According to the Regulations, Common Specifications (CS) can now also contribute more detailed presumptions of conformity for certain product groups, especially in the clinical area, or even be binding for Annex XVI products! The lists with the titles of the harmonised European standards which contain presumptions of conformity for one or both Regulations are published 1-2 times a year in the Official Journal of the EU under the heading of the Regulation concerned. The standards themselves are available (in the desired language) from the national standards institutes of the Member States, generally for a fee. Common specifications will be published as Implementing Acts of the COM in the Official Journal of the EU and will also be available via links on the COM website (medical devices sector; see link list).

5.1 Risk Management System (RMS): based on a **risk management plan**;

the manufacturer must introduce, implement, document and update a risk management system and operate it as a life cycle process under its QMS and systematically keep it up-to-date[194]. This RMS must perform the following (see Fig.15):

☐ Define and document a risk management plan for each MD/IVD;

---

[192] Except those for harmonized symbols and identification colors

[193] E.g. those of ISO or IEC, which may refer to essential principles of the IMDRF, instead of to the GSPR of the European regulations; in case of doubt please perform a gap analysis to the GSPR and clarify with your NB!

[194] See also EN ISO 14971, especially when harmonised to MDR/IVDR. For even more detail also look at: ISO Technical Report TR 24971: Medical devices — Guidance on the application of ISO 14971

- □ identify known and foreseeable hazards for each product (if possible, by type, severity, probability);
- □ assess and evaluate the risks of the MD/IVD (if possible, according to type, severity, probability), when used as intended and under reasonably foreseeable misuse;
- □ eliminate or minimise the identified risks in accordance with the risk control principles (see below);
- □ Risks are to be minimized as far as possible, as is possible without negative effects on the benefit/risk ratio[195];
- □ All known and foreseeable risks, and any undesirable side-effects, shall be minimised and be acceptable when weighed against the evaluated benefits to the patient and/or user arising from the achieved performance of the device during normal conditions of use[196];
- □ Assess the impact of information from the manufacturing phase and PMS on hazards and risks, as well as on the overall benefit/risk ratio and risk acceptance, and
- □ adjust the risk control measures in accordance with the risk control principles on the basis of the above assessment.

The **risk control measures** for design and manufacture follow these principles:
- □ they comply with the safety principles, considering the generally recognised state of the art,
- □ Risk management in risk reduction aims at the acceptability of
  - ○ residual risks associated with each hazard, as well as of the
  - ○ overall risk

---

[195] See Annex I.I.2 of both Regulations
[196] MDR/IVDR: Annex I.I.8.

When selecting the most appropriate solutions, the following **order of risk control measures** must be followed:

1. eliminate or minimise risks as far as possible through **safe design and manufacture**;
2. if necessary, take **appropriate protective measures**, including **alarms**, for risks that cannot be excluded;
3. provide **safety information** (warnings, cautions, contraindications) and, where appropriate, **training** for users; manufacturers shall inform users of any residual risks.

To exclude or reduce **risks due to use errors**, the manufacturer must consider (incl. usability[197]):

☐ Risks due to ergonomic features of the MD/IVD and the application environment (product design geared to the safety of the patient) and
☐ the technical knowledge, experience, training and further education, if necessary, application environment, health and physical condition of the intended users (laypersons, specialists, handicapped persons or other user-oriented product design).

For the minimization or elimination of risks, especially concerning Chapter II of Annexes I the following principle has to be considered:

Annex I.I.2. of MDR/IVDR: *The requirement in this Annex to reduce risks as far as possible means the reduction of risks as far as possible without adversely affecting the benefit- risk ratio.*

(Harmonized) standards will support and guide your risk management system build-up:

EN ISO 14971: Medical devices — Application of risk management to medical devices

ISO/TR 24971: Medical devices — Guidance on the application of ISO 14971

---

[197] See also EN IEC 62366-1: Medical devices — Application of usability engineering to medical devices

A lot of more specific standards are also based on a risk management concept, applied to specific areas, e.g. EN ISO 10993-series, EN ISO 18562-series, EN ISO 22442-series, (in the series, usually Part 1 addresses specifically risk management even in the title), ISO 22367 etc.

Fig. 15 MDR-IVDR: Risk Management

Risk-Management acc. to Annex I MDR/IVDR			
Risk-Management-System	Continuous iterative process over life-cycle, under QMS!	establish, implement document, maintain	regular systematic updating
Risk-Management-Plan	for each MD/IVD	establish document	
Hazards	known + foreseeable; associated with each MD/IVD	Identify analyse	type, severity, probability
Risks	during intended use and reasonably foreseeable misuse	estimate evaluate	type, severity, probability
Risk-control	Annex I.Section I.4	Section I.2: eliminate, reduce AFAP. Reduction of risks as far as possible without adversely affecting the benefit –risk ratio	3 – Hierarchy of Risk-Control* 2-Use Errors**
Continuous evaluation of information	from **production phase** + **PMS**	Evaluation of impact on:	hazards/risks, overall risk, benefit-risk ratio + risk acceptability
Risk Control adapted	Annex I.Section I.4	eliminate, reduce risks AFAP	3 – Hierarchy of Risk-Control* 2-Use Errors**

*3-Hierarchy Risk-Control: Annex I.I.4:
1. Inherent safe design and manufacture
2. Protection measures, incl Alarms
3. Safety Information, poss. User Training

**Protection against Use Errors due to:
1. Ergonomic Features, Environment
2. User characteristics (lay, professional, disabled ...)

Fig. 16 Annex I: 4-Step Procedure

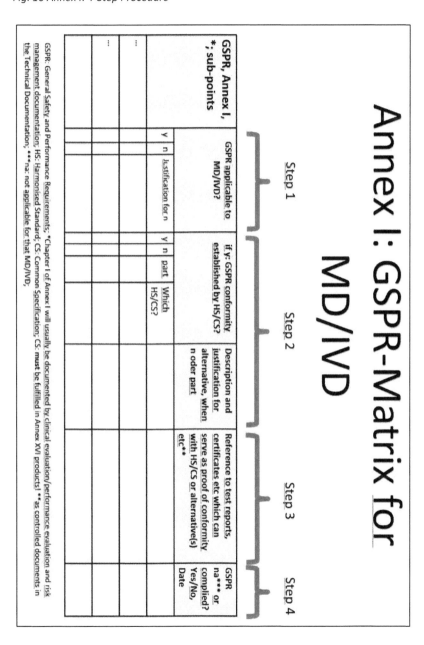

Annex I: GSPR-Matrix for MD/IVD

GSPR, Annex I, *, sub-points	GSPR applicable to MD/IVD?			if y: GSPR conformity established by HS/CS?				Description and justification for alternative, when n oder part	Reference to test reports, certificates etc which can serve as proof of conformity with HS/CS or alternative(s) etc**	GSPR na*** or complied? Yes/No, Date
	y	n	Justification for n	y	n	part	Which HS/CS?			
...										
...										

Step 1 — Step 2 — Step 3 — Step 4

GSPR: General Safety and Performance Requirements; *Chapter I of Annex I will usually be documented by clinical evaluation/ performance evaluation and risk management documentation; HS: Harmonised Standard; CS: Common Specification; CS: **must** be fulfilled in Annex XVI products! **as controlled documents in the Technical Documentation; ***na: not applicable for that MD/IVD;

5.2. Matrix of General Safety and Performance Requirements

Fig. 16 shows how the General Safety and Performance Requirements (GSPR; especially Chap. II and III of Annex I and their sub-items) can be systematically processed in 4 steps by means of harmonised standards and common specifications or alternative solutions. **Chapter I of Annex I** are to be processed in the **MDR** relying on the <u>clinical evaluation and risk management system</u> and be documented in detail in those processes; Chapter I of Annex I and Chapter I.II.9.1. of **IVDR** are processed relying on the <u>performance evaluation and the risk management system</u> and the relevant documentation.

For the systematic processing of the requirements especially of **Chapter II and III of Annex I** and their documentation, it is recommended to create a **GSPR matrix**[198] (lines: individually listed GSPR including their respective sub-items! Columns: Steps of examination, testing and verification procedures and their results): see Fig. 16:

Step 1: Does the GSPR or its sub-item apply to my MD/IVD: yes - no? If no, a short explanation may be recommended (also for verification by the NB or CA[199])
Step 2: if yes in step 1: Do I comply with this GSPR or sub-item completely or partially (yes - partly) or not (no) by following a harmonised European standard (HS; see Annex Z with the specific presumptions of conformity) or a Common Specification (CS)? If the answer is partly or no, a presentation and justification of the alternative way chosen to fulfil the relevant GSPR or sub-items must be provided instead of the HS or CS. Note for the MDR: Annex XVI-MD must comply with the applicable CS!
Step 3: Detailed references to the concrete evidence, test reports, test results, certificates, etc. for compliance with the GSPR or sub-items, either in whole or in part by means of the procedures described in the HS or CS or the alternative solutions for the HS or parts thereof set out and justified by the manufacturer. These verifications, test reports, test results, certificates, etc. must be traceable as controlled documents under the manufacturer's QMS and stored in the technical documentation.

---

[198] See a GSPR matrix template for MDR: Annex I in WORD format: MDCG 2021-8: Clinical investigation application/notification documents (Annex: Checklist of general safety and performance requirements, Standards, common specifications and scientific advice)
[199] CA Competent Authority

Step 4: Here the concluding assessment is made as to whether the corresponding GSPR or the sub-item has been processed in conformity with the respective Regulation (either the GSPR does not apply to the MD/IVD at all or the required evidence could be provided in accordance with HS/CS or alternative solution), possibly with the date of this assessment.

Fig. 17 MDR: Annex I Overview

MDR Annex I

I. General Requirements

Clinical Evaluation	Risk-Management

II. Requirements regarding Design and Manufacturer

10. Chem., physical., biological properties
11. Infection and microbial contamination
12. Medicinal products and other substances
13. Materials of biological origin
14. Construction and interaction with environment
15. Diagnostic or measuring function
16. Protection against radiation
17. Electronic programmable systems, Software
18. Active devices
19. Active implantable devices
20. Mechanical and thermal risks
21. Risks by supplying energy or substances
22. Risks by lay persons' use

III. Information to be supplied with Device

23.1. General requirements regarding the information
23.2. Label
23.3. Sterile packaging
23.4. Instructions for use

5.3 Important changes[200] to the General Safety and Performance Requirements for MDs in Annex I

See overview in Fig. 17.

Chapter I (General requirements) of Annex I centers on **clinical evaluation**[201] and the **risk management system**[202].

Chap. II and Chap. III of Annex I of the MDR contain more specific aspects of risk management and performance:

MDR: Annex I, Chapter II:

Section 10: Chemical, physical and biological properties:

The main focus here is on the risks and risk minimisation through the selection of materials, surface properties and substances used for the MD, including the risks from released substances or particles, including abrasion, degradation products, processing and process residues, with regard to:

- compatibility with biological tissues, cells or body fluids,
    - concerning biocompatibility and toxicological safety[203] (toxicokinetics, toxicodynamics)
    - Type of tissue exposed and duration and frequency of exposure,
    - Properties and size of particles that can be introduced into the body, including nanomaterials,
    - compliance with validated biophysical and other models, if applicable,
- Mechanical properties (e.g. strength, ductility, fracture resistance, wear and fatigue resistance),
- Surface properties and finish,
- Compliance with chemical/physical specifications[204],

---

[200] Compared to the previous Directives!

[201] see chapter 7 in this book

[202] see chapter 5.1 in this book

[203] See specifically (harmonised) standard series EN ISO 10993 ‚Biological evaluation of medical devices' EN ISO 18562 'Biocompatibility Evaluation of Breathing Gas Pathway Devices' and chapter 5.4. (Preclinical Evaluation) in this book

[204] See here EN ISO 10993-18 and 19 for reference

- Compatibility with materials, substances, including gases, drugs with which they may come into contact during intended use,
- Compatibility of the different parts of the MD, especially within implants,
- Flammability,
- Unintentional penetration/ingress of substances into the MD.

This section is particularly important for the **preclinical evaluation of MDs**[205], see chapter V.4. below!

Section 11: Infection and microbial contamination

In accordance with the new protection regulations against **needle-stick injuries** in occupational safety, risks due to unintended cuts and pricks must be minimized as far as possible and appropriate in terms of design[206]. Section 11.5 now explicitly refers to **validated sterilization procedures**[207].

Section 12: Products containing a substance considered as a medicinal product and products consisting of substances or combinations of substances absorbed by the human body or distributed locally in the body[208]

12.1: Quality, safety and benefits of pharmaceutical components in an ancillary function shall be verified by analogy to the methods in Annex I to Directive 2001/83/EEC on medicinal products.

Specific requirements, including dossier requirements for consultation procedures can be found in EMA-Guidance[209]

---

[205] See chapter 5.4. in this book for preclinical evaluation of MDs

[206] A lot of harmonized standards are already available in that respect

[207] See e.g. examples of the wealth of harmonized standards available in chapter 1.4.4. in this book

[208] See EMA's homepage on interaction issues between pharmaceutical sector and medical device/IVD sector: https://www.ema.europa.eu/en/human-regulatory/overview/medical-devices

[209] E.g. European Medicines Agency recommendation on the procedural aspects and dossier requirements for the consultation of the European Medicines Agency by a notified body on

12.2: the substances or combinations of substances mentioned must, where appropriate and limited to the aspects not covered by the MDR, meet the requirements set out in Annex I to Directive 2001/83/EC with regard to the evaluation of absorption, distribution, metabolism, excretion, local tolerance, toxicity, interactions with other medical devices, medicinal products or other substances and possible adverse reactions. Please consult here also the EMA homepage, as shown above!

Please also note the possibility of a consultation procedure according to Annex IX.II.5.2 and 5.4., possibly Annex IX.II.6, respectively Annex X.6 and Annex XI.A.8 or XI.B.16!

Section 13: Devices incorporating materials of biological origin

13.1: For devices manufactured utilising derivatives of tissues or cells of **human origin** which are non-viable or are rendered non-viable[210] covered by this Regulation in accordance with point (g) of Article 1(6), the following shall apply:

(a) donation, procurement and testing of the tissues and cells shall be done in accordance with Directive 2004/23/EC ('Tissue Directive');

(b) processing, preservation and any other handling of those tissues and cells or their derivatives shall be carried out so as to provide safety for patients, users and, where applicable, other persons. In particular, safety with regard to viruses and other transmissible agents shall be addressed by appropriate methods of sourcing and by implementation of validated methods of elimination or inactivation in the course of the manufacturing process;

(c) the traceability system for those devices shall be complementary and compatible with the traceability and data protection requirements laid down in Directive 2004/23/EC and in Directive 2002/98/EC.

---

an ancillary medicinal substance or an ancillary human blood derivative incorporated in a medical device or active implantable medical device: https://www.ema.europa.eu/en/documents/regulatory-procedural-guideline/ema-recommendation-procedural-aspects-dossier-requirements-consultation-ema-notified-body-ancillary_en.pdf

[210] MDR: Art. 2 (16) 'non-viable' means having no potential for metabolism or multiplication;

Note: in 13.1. a serious content/editorial error of the MDR:
The provisions a)-c) would of course also have to apply to the non-viable an-
cillary components of human origin in MD according to Art. 1 (10), 1st sub-
paragraph!

13.2 For devices manufactured utilising tissues or cells of **animal origin**, or their derivatives, which are non-viable or rendered non-viable[211] the following shall apply[212]:
(a) where feasible taking into account the animal species, tissues and cells of animal origin, or their derivatives, shall originate from animals that have been subjected to veterinary controls that are adapted to the intended use of the tissues. Information on the geographical origin of the animals shall be retained by manufacturers;
(b) sourcing, processing, preservation, testing and handling of tissues, cells and substances of animal origin, or their derivatives, shall be carried out so as to provide safety for patients, users and, where applicable, other persons. In particular, safety with regard to viruses and other transmissible agents shall be addressed by implementation of validated methods of elimination or viral inactivation in the course of the manufacturing process, except when the use of such methods would lead to unacceptable degradation compromising the clinical benefit of the device;
(c) in the case of devices manufactured utilising tissues or cells of animal origin, or their derivatives, as referred to in Regulation (EU) No 722/2012[213] the particular requirements laid down in that Regulation shall apply.

....

---

[211] MDR: Art. 2 (16) 'non-viable' means having no potential for metabolism or multiplication;
[212] See also EN ISO series 22442 Medical devices utilizing animal tissues and their derivatives
[213] Commission Regulation (EU) No 722/2012 of 8 August 2012 concerning particular requirements as regards the requirements laid down in Council Directives 90/385/EEC and 93/42/EEC with respect to active implantable medical devices and medical devices manufactured utilising tissues of animal origin Please note that this Regulation under Directives 93/42/EEC and 90/385/EEC is now also an implementing Regulation under the MDR.

> Section 17: Electronic Programmable Systems - Devices that incorporate electronic programmable systems and Software that are devices in themselves[214]

There has been a significant expansion and deepening of the requirements here[215]:

17.1. Devices that incorporate electronic programmable systems, including software, or software that are devices in themselves, shall be designed to **ensure repeatability, reliability and performance** in line with their intended use. In the event of a **single fault condition**, appropriate means shall be adopted to eliminate or reduce as far as possible consequent risks or impairment of performance.

17.2. For devices that incorporate software or for software that are devices in themselves, the software shall be developed and manufactured in acordance with the state of the art taking into account the **principles of development life cycle[216], risk management, including information security, verification and validation**.

17.3. Software referred to in this Section that is intended to be used in combination with mobile computing platforms shall be designed and manufactured taking into account the specific features of the **mobile platform** (e.g. size and contrast ratio of the screen) and the **external factors related to their use** (e.g. varying environment as regards level of light or noise).

17.4. Manufacturers shall set out minimum requirements concerning **hardware, IT networks characteristics and IT security measures[217], including protection against unauthorised access**, necessary to run the software as intended.

---

[214] See MDCG 2019-11: Qualification and classification of software - Regulation (EU) 2017/745 and Regulation (EU) 2017/746, which differentiates 'MDSW-Medical Device Software' and 'Software driving or influencing the use of a medical device'. In IMDRF MDSW is called SaMD: Software as a MD

[215] See also MDCG 2019-11: Qualification and classification of software - Regulation (EU) 2017/745 and Regulation (EU) 2017/746

[216] See EN IEC 62304 Medical device software - Software life-cycle processes

[217] See MDCG 2019-16, rev. 1: 'Guidance on cybersecurity for medical devices' and MDCG 2020-1: 'Guidance on clinical evaluation (MDR) / Performance evaluation (IVDR) of medical device software'

.....

Section 19: Specific requirements for active implantable devices:

Due to the integration of Directive 90/385/EEC into the MDR, relevant requirements for active implantable MD had to be transferred from Annex I of AIMDD to Annex I of the MDR as well.

In particular, risks in connection with **energy sources** (especially insulation, leakage currents, and heating of products), with **medical interventions** (e.g. defibrillation, electrosurgery), with **lack of maintenance or calibration**, the **compatibility with substances** which they are to administer, and the **reliability of the energy source** must also be taken into account.

After all, protective measures concerning special requirements for the identification of products and, if necessary, their components, are necessary.

It shall be possible to read the identification code they have to bear without surgical operation[218].

....

Section 22: Protection against the risks posed by lay use

This section is new for medical devices (was previously only available in IVD Directive 98/79/EC). However, the increasing spread of MD for lay persons also requires special requirements here[219]:

These products must be designed and manufactured in such a way that they can fulfil their intended purpose, taking into account the skills and possibilities of lay persons and the effects of the fluctuations in the procedures and environment normally to be expected of lay persons. The information and instructions provided by the manufacturer must be easily understandable and applicable to lay persons.

MDs for lay use shall be designed and manufactured in such a way that

- it is guaranteed that the product can be used safely and faultlessly by the intended user in all operating phases - if necessary, after appropriate training and/or information,

---

[218] See also: MDCG 2019-8 v2: Guidance document implant card on the application of Article 18 Regulation (EU) 2017/745 on medical devices
[219] See also EN 62366-1: Medical devices - Application of usability engineering to medical devices

- the risks caused by unintended cuts or pricks, such as needle stick injuries, are reduced as far as possible and appropriate; and
- the risk of error by the intended user in the handling of the device or, if applicable, incorrect interpretation of the results by the intended user is kept as low as possible.

- Devices for lay use shall, where appropriate, be provided with a procedure for the lay person to verify, at the time of use, that the device will work as intended by the MF and, where appropriate, to warn if the device has failed to provide a valid result.

MDR: Annex I, Chapter III:

Section 23: Requirements for the Information
provided with the device

This section is again extremely detailed for a New Approach Act.

Section 23.1. deals with the general requirements for the provision of information in labelling and instructions for use, which take account of further developments in this area; The focus is on the precise identification of MDs and manufacturers and the safety and performance information relevant to users, patients and third parties.

(a) The medium, format, content, legibility, and location of the label and understandability of instructions for use shall be appropriate to the particular device, its intended purpose and the technical knowledge, experience, education or training of the intended user(s).

(b) The information required on the label shall be provided on the device itself. If this is not practicable or appropriate, some or all of the information may appear on the packaging for each unit, and/or on the packaging of multiple devices.

(c) Labels shall be provided in a human-readable format and may be supplemented by machine-readable information, such as radio-frequency identification ('RFID') or bar codes.

(d) Instructions for use shall be provided together with devices. By way of exception, instructions for use shall not be required for class I and class IIa devices if such devices can be used safely without any such instructions and unless otherwise provided for elsewhere in this Section.

(e) Where multiple devices are supplied to a single user and/or location, a single copy of the instructions for use may be provided if so agreed by the purchaser who in any case may request further copies to be provided free of charge.

(f) Instructions for use may be provided to the user in non-paper format (e.g. electronic) to the extent, and only under the conditions, set out in Regulation (EU) No 207/2012 or in any subsequent implementing rules adopted pursuant to this Regulation.

(g) Residual risks which are required to be communicated to the user and/or other person shall be included as limitations, contra-indications, precautions or warnings in the information supplied by the manufacturer.

(h) Where appropriate, the information supplied by the manufacturer shall take the form of internationally recognised symbols. **Any symbol or identification colour used shall (=must) conform to the harmonised standards or CS.** In areas for which no harmonised standards or CS exist, the symbols and colours shall be described in the documentation supplied with the device.

Sections 23.2 (**labelling**), 23.3 (**sterile packaging**) and 23.4 (**instructions for use**)[220]: You should work these sections through meticulously as a checklist when designing the respective identification drawings and instructions for use, where applicable in individual cases. In particular, relevant clinical, hygienic and risk-relevant aspects were presented in much more detail. The labelling now has its own requirements for sterile packaging.

Please note the following: Commission Implementing Regulation (EU) 2021/2226 of 14 December 2021 laying down rules for the application of Regulation (EU) 2017/745 of the European Parliament and of the Council as regards **electronic instructions for use of medical devices**[221]

Further information to be provided for certain high-risk MDs includes, for implants and Class III MDs, the **Summary on Safety and Clinical Performance (SSCP)**[222] ac-

---

[220] See also ISO 15223-1: Medical devices — Symbols to be used with medical device labels, labelling and information to be supplied — Part 1: General requirements (harmonised European symbols and identification colors will be binding!); see also: ISO 20417 Medical devices — Information to be supplied by the manufacturer; and labelling and/or IFU-elements in specific product (group) standards.

[221] https://eur-lex.europa.eu/eli/reg_impl/2021/2226/oj

[222] See MDCG 2019-9: Summary of safety and clinical performance

cording to Art. 32 (see Chapter VI Clinical Evaluation) and for certain implants, with exceptions, the relevant **implant information** according to Art. 18 of MDR[223].

5.4. Preclinical Evaluation of MDs

acc. to MDR: Annex I and VII and (highly recommended) EN ISO series 10993 'Biological evaluation of medical devices', see Tab. 7-8.

For specific applications the following standards may also be useful: e.g. ISO EN 18562 series on 'Biocompatibility evaluation of breathing gas pathways in healthcare applications', see Tab. 9 and ISO 7405 'Dentistry — Evaluation of biocompatibility of medical devices used in dentistry'. Some product specific standards may also contain specific provisions for preclinical evaluation.

'Preclinical evaluation of medical devices' is used here synonymously with 'biological evaluation of medical devices' and with 'biocompatibility evaluation of medical devices'.

Preclinical evaluation is one of the life-cycle processes of the MDR, to be planned, implemented and documented by the manufacturer under his QMS and in close connection with his risk management system. MDR describes this process indirectly in its Annex VII.4.5.4., when requesting how NBs will have to look at it in the conformity assessment of manufacturers.

The process of preclinical evaluation is here developed in line with MDR and EN ISO 10993 acc. to the general scheme used in MDR for life-cycle processes under a QMS. The process has to be carried out by/with the help of experienced and knowledgeable professionals via (scientific) literature review[224] and collection of other valid biological data and planning and performing necessary biological and chemical tests[225].

The best starting point to plan, implement and document a preclinical evaluation is EN ISO 10993: 'Biological evaluation of medical devices — Part 1: Evaluation and testing within a risk management process':

---

[223] See MDCG 2019-8 v2: Guidance document implant card on the application of Article 18 Regulation (EU) 2017/745 on medical devices
[224] See EN ISO 10993-1: Annex C
[225] See survey in EN ISO 10993-!: clause 6.3. and EN ISO 10993-series

1. establish a **plan for the activity** with a frame guiding it
- from the Material characterisation of MD (chemical, physical) with direct or indirect body contact,
- categorize the MD by nature and duration of body contact and selection of Endpoints for necessary biological risk evaluation,
- towards the objectives of the exercise:
  - o identification and assessment of potential biological hazards and related risks;
  - o determining acceptability of biological risks against possible alternatives and with a view to the overall B/R-Profile of the MD,

2. collect relevant data systematically and generate data if necessary, when identifying data gaps, which will have to be closed (e.g. by appropriate chemical or biological tests);

3. evaluate these data by appraisal/analysis and draw conclusions on the acceptability of results towards the objectives;

4. compile a report on the process performed and its results;

5. continue the life-cycle process on systematically collected new data (from production and post-production phase; e.g. changes, unexpected adverse effects, effects after multiple reuse, previously unknown interactions or uses etc.) with new data evaluation and update of the report, together with necessary conclusions on possible/necessary CAPAs and improvements or re-evaluations.

Preclinical evaluation steps:
Preclinical evaluation should start with a **preclinical evaluation plan**. The plan should include the arrangements for the steps to be performed in preclinical evaluation in order to be in line with the risk management plan acc. to EN ISO 14971. These steps will contain at least the following elements:

a) **Material characterization** with a **detailed description of the MD, its configuration, composition and its intended purpose/use, with a view to possible direct and indirect body contact**:

Composition will encompass a **detailed specification and verification of qualitative and quantitative data of materials used** in manufacture, construction, processes (e.g. sterilisation), finish, packaging etc. where these materials concerned might come into direct or indirect contact with the human body:

Material characterization[226]:
— the material(s) of manufacture;
— intended additives, process contaminants and residues;
— substances released in normal use;
— degradation products from normal use that might pass into the patient;
— other components and their interactions in the final medical device, part or accessory;
— the performance and characteristics of the final medical device, part or accessory;
— physical characteristics of the final medical device, part or accessory including, but not limited to, porosity, particle size and shape;
— the effects of any hygienic processing steps required before use or re-use, if applicable.

Aspects of **configuration** of the MD will describe e.g. size, geometry, shape and relative arrangement of the parts of the MD, surface properties, components and their interaction etc).

These descriptions usually will include a **chemical characterization of materials** in direct or indirect contact with the human body (preferably acc. to Part 18 of EN ISO 10993) and a **Physico-chemical, morphological and topographical characterization of materials,** (as described acc. to Part 19 of ISO/TR 10993).

---

b) Of particular concern will be the **potential release[227] of substances and/or particles from the MD** and its materials during the life cycle of the MD, esp. during its use.

Direct or indirect contact with the human body of these may constitute specific problems for the assessment of biological safety, the more if this will

---

[226] The extent of material characterisation is of course dependent on the risk of MDs, e.g. might be less with a class I MD with short duration contact only to intact skin; Example given here is of ISO 18562-1: Biocompatibility evaluation of breathing gas pathways in healthcare applications — Part 1: Evaluation and testing within a risk management process
[227] Quality and quantity

lead to internal exposure. This release of substances/particles may refer to potential e.g. leachables, degradation products, wear particles, process residues (e.g. after EO sterilisation), possible residual process aids or additives during manufacture, monomeric/oligomeric residues after incomplete polymerisation, manufacturing residues, corrosion products, nanomaterials[228]. Potential for degradation may exist under conditions of manufacture, sterilisation, transport, storage and use (incl. reuse). Part 9 of EN ISO 10993 may help here with its 'Framework for identification and quantification of potential degradation products'; to be specified further, if applicable to the specific MD, by Parts 13, 14 or 15 of EN ISO 10993 for 'Identification and quantification of degradation products from polymeric MDs, or ceramics or from metals and alloys'. Also EN ISO 10993-18 will be important here, with its information on analytics.

Part 22 of EN ISO 10993: 'Guidance on nanomaterials will be particularly important for this product group.

c) a clear specification of the **intended purpose/use of the MD**[229] will be **particularly important to categorize the nature and duration of contact of the MD and its materials with the human body.**

EN ISO 10993-Part 1 provides a matrix system for such categorization, which establishes various categories, types of tissue contact and duration of contact and correlates it to the **proposed endpoints** of biological risk evaluation[230], which will have to be discussed for the MD in question.

Categories and contact tissues[231] will be:

Surface contacting MDs, with
skin (e.g. electrodes, external prostheses, fixation tapes, bandages),
mucosal membranes (e.g. contact lenses, urinary catheters, endoscopes etc) and

---

[228] Quantity of release (potential for internal exposure) of nanomaterials will be particularly important for the classification of MDs acc. to Ann. VIII, Rule 19

[229] Clear description of intended purpose/use of the MD must be consistent over all relevant documents and processes, like Technical documentation (TD), clinical evaluation and risk management under the MDR.

[230] See chapter 5 (Categorization of medical devices) and Annex A (Endpoints to be addressed in a biological risk assessment) of EN ISO 10993-1. Table A.1. (Endpoints to be addressed in a biological risk assessment) provides an excellent survey on biological evaluation of MD!

[231] See EN ISO 10993-1: chapter 5.2. and Annex A, Table A.1.

breaches or compromised surfaces (e.g. dressings, occlusive patches for ulcers, burns and granulation tissue)

Externally communicating MDs, with the following tissue contacts:

Blood path, indirect (e.g. administration sets, transfer sets, blood administration sets)

Tissue/bone/dentin (laparoscopes, arthroscopes, draining systems, dental filling materials) means

direct or indirect (e.g. serve as a conduit to deliver fluids to these tissues) contact with these tissues

Circulating blood (e.g. intravascular catheters, oxygenators, dialysers, haemoadsorbents)

Implant MDs

Tissue, bone (e.g. orthopedic pins, plates, replacement joints, bone cements)

Blood (e.g. heart valves, vascular grafts, ventricular assist devices)

Categorization by duration of contact will be:

- *Limited exposure* with cumulative sum of single, multiple or repeated contact duration **up to 24h**
  There is also a special category for *transitory-contacting MDs*, for very short contact times of less than 1 min (e.g lancets, hypodermic needles) which would normally not require biocompatibility testing, unless coated or with lubricants.
- *Prolonged exposure* cumulative contact duration **between 24h and 30d**
- *Long-term exposure* cumulative contact time **> 30d**

d) determination of exposure qualitatively and quantitatively through various routes

(EN ISO 10993, Parts 9, 13, 14, 15 and 22 will be of help here, if necessary also Part 16 for 'Toxicokinetic study design for degradation products and leachables'; Part 18 will again be helpful here).

e) **selection of endpoints** of biological risk assessment with rationale[232], which will be assessed during the further steps of preclinical evaluation

f) **assess selected endpoints**

with the help of scientific preclinical literature[233] and other available and

---

[232] For inclusion or omission, e.g. against Table A.1. in EN ISO 10993-1, Annex A; specific MD might also need specific endpoints (e.g. for nephrotoxicity, thrombogenicity)

[233] See EN ISO 10993-1: Annex C

valid biocompatibility data, e.g. of equivalent MDs or reliance on presumptions of conformity from harmonised standards or Common Specifications followed by a gap analysis of necessary biocompatibility data; demonstration of compliance is necessary with regard to the relevant requirements in Annex I.II., section 10 (Chemical, physical and biological properties), with a discussion and justification of the chosen solutions for substances, materials, surface properties etc. from a risk/benefit point of view against possible alternatives. Requirements of section 12 (Medicinal products and substances/substance combinations) and section 13 of Annex I.II. (Medical devices with materials of biological origin) may also be of concern for preclinical evaluation.

g) **perform biological testing**[234] to close the gaps identified

h) determine whether - from all data retrieved by biological literature search and biological testing – **biological safety** over relevant endpoints has been established[235] and overall B/R-profile is acceptable against possible alternatives and residual biological risks are acceptable against the overall B/R-profile of the MD.

i) compile a **preclinical evaluation report** with details of the process over its steps, summary of biological data retrieved, of assessments performed and results with regard to biological safety and demonstration of acceptability against alternatives; qualification of preclinical evaluators shall be displayed.

---

[234] Acc. to EN ISO 10993-1: clause 6.3. and Annex B.4.2.; Good Laboratory Practice (GLP) will be a preference. GLP studies are carried out to defined quality standards in laboratories that are accredited in line with an internationally implemented governmental scheme. Typically studies will be conducted under a laboratory quality system compliant to ISO/IEC 17025 or an equivalent standard (EN ISO 10993-1, clause B.4.5.2)

[235] E.g. with the help of EN ISO 10993-17: 'Establishment of allowable limits for leachable substances, Thresholds of Toxicological concern (TTC), and state of the art toxicological science/expertise, look also at EN ISO 10993-18 and ISO TS 21726: Biological evaluation of medical devices — Application of the threshold of toxicological concern (TTC) for assessing biocompatibility of medical device constituents

j) **continue biological evaluation over the life-cycle of the MD** under consideration of changes[236] encountered, unexpected adverse effects, and other indications from PMS or PMCF and update the preclinical evaluation report accordingly.

Tab. 7 Survey of EN ISO 10993-1 for basic orientation

Clause 4 'General principles for the biological evaluation of medical devices';
Clause 5, 'Categorization of medical devices' (MDs are categorized acc. to nature and duration of body contact);
Clause 6 'biocompatibility assessment process';
Clause 7 'Evaluation of biological assessment data and overall assessment of biological safety';
Annex A, 'Endpoints to be addressed in a biological risk assessment';
See here in particular Table A.1 'Endpoints to be addressed in a biological risk assessment'. In the table you will find a matrix of the endpoints to be discussed for the various categories of MDs in the biological risk evaluation;
Annex B 'Guidance on the conduct of biological evaluation within a risk management process';
Annex C: "Suggested procedure for literature review".

Tab. 8 Survey of EN ISO 10993-series

ISO 10993-1, Biological evaluation of medical devices — Part 1: Evaluation and testing within a risk management process.
ISO 10993-2, Biological evaluation of medical devices — Part 2: Animal welfare requirements
ISO 10993-3, Biological evaluation of medical devices — Part 3: Tests for genotoxicity, carcinogenicity and reproductive toxicity
ISO 10993-4, Biological evaluation of medical devices — Part 4: Selection of tests for interactions with blood

---

[236] Acc. to clause 4.9. of EN ISO 10993-1: The biological risk assessment of materials or final products shall be re-evaluated if any of the following occur:
a) any change in the source or in the specification of the materials used in the manufacture of the product;
b) any change in the formulation, processing, primary packaging or sterilization of the product;
c) any change in the manufacturer's instructions or expectations concerning storage, e.g. changes in shelf life and/or transport;
d) any change in the intended use of the product;
e) any evidence that the product can produce adverse biological effects when used in humans.

ISO 10993-5, Biological evaluation of medical devices — Part 5: Tests for in vitro cytotoxicity

ISO 10993-6, Biological evaluation of medical devices — Part 6: Tests for local effects after implantation

ISO 10993-7, Biological evaluation of medical devices — Part 7: Ethylene oxide sterilization residuals

ISO 10993-9, Biological evaluation of medical devices — Part 9: Framework for identification and quantification of potential degradation products

ISO 10993-10, Biological evaluation of medical devices — Part 10: Tests for irritation and skin sensitization

ISO 10993-11, Biological evaluation of medical devices — Part 11: Tests for systemic toxicity

ISO 10993-12, Biological evaluation of medical devices — Part 12: Sample preparation and reference materials

ISO 10993-13, Biological evaluation of medical devices — Part 13: Identification and quantification of degradation products from polymeric medical devices

ISO 10993-14, Biological evaluation of medical devices — Part 14: Identification and quantification of degradation products from ceramics

ISO 10993-15, Biological evaluation of medical devices — Part 15: Identification and quantification of degradation products from metals and alloys

ISO 10993-16, Biological evaluation of medical devices — Part 16: Toxicokinetic study design for degradation products and leachables

ISO 10993-17, Biological evaluation of medical devices — Part 17: Establishment of allowable limits for leachable substances

ISO 10993-18, Biological evaluation of medical devices — Part 18: Chemical characterization of materials

ISO/TR 10993-19, Biological evaluation of medical devices — Part 19: Physico-chemical, morphological and topographical characterization of materials

ISO/TS 10993-20, Biological evaluation of medical devices — Part 20: Principles and methods for immunotoxicology testing of medical devices

ISO/TR 10993-22: Biological evaluation of medical devices — Part 22: Guidance on nanomaterials

Tab. 9 Survey of EN ISO 18562-series

ISO 18562-1, Biocompatibility evaluation of breathing gas pathways in healthcare applications — Part 1: Evaluation and testing within a risk management process

ISO 18562-2, Biocompatibility evaluation of breathing gas pathways in healthcare applications — Part 2: Tests for emissions of particulate matter

ISO 18562-3, Biocompatibility evaluation of breathing gas pathways in healthcare applications — Part 3: Tests for emissions of volatile organic compounds (VOCs)

A significant new point of preclinical evaluation addressed in MDR in this section 10 of Annex I of MDR has been:

Risks from CMR[237] substances and endocrine disrupters (ED)[238]:

To avert these risks, new, explicit provisions have been added to the MDR which provide for an obligation to justify and set precautionary measures for the following MDs:

MD or components or materials contained therein which

- are applied invasively and come into direct contact with the body,
- (re-)administer or withdraw medicinal products, body fluids or other substances, including gases, from the body, or
- transport or store such medicinal products, body fluids or other substances, including gases, which are (re-)administered to the body,

shall only <u>contain the following substances</u> in a concentration that is above 0,1 % weight by weight (w/w) where justified pursuant to Section 10.4.2:

(a) **substances which are carcinogenic, mutagenic or toxic to reproduction ('CMR'),** of category 1A or 1B, in accordance with Part 3 of Annex VI to Regulation (EC) No 1272/2008 of the European Parliament and of the Council[239], or

(b) **substances having endocrine-disrupting properties** for which there is scientific evidence of probable serious effects to human health and which are identified either in accordance with the procedure set out in Article 59 of Regulation (EC) No 1907/2006 of the European Parliament and of the Council[240] or, once a delegated act has been adopted by the Commission

---

[237] CMR: carcinogenic, mutagenic or reproduction toxic
[238] Endocrine disruptors: hormonally active substances
[239] Regulation (EC) No 1272/2008 of the European Parliament and of the Council of 16 December 2008 on classification, labelling and packaging of substances and mixtures, amending and repealing Directives 67/548/EEC and 1999/45/EC, and amending Regulation (EC) No 1907/2006 (OJ L 353, 31.12.2008, p. 1);
[240] Regulation (EC) No 1907/2006 of the European Parliament and of the Council of 18 December 2006 concerning the Registration, Evaluation, Authorisation and Restriction of Chemicals (REACH) (OJ L 396, 30.12.2006, p. 1);

pursuant to the first subparagraph of Article 5(3) of Regulation (EU) No 528/2012 of the European Parliament and the Council[241], in accordance with the criteria that are relevant to human health amongst the criteria established therein. The justification for the presence of these substances must be based on:

(a) an analysis and estimation of the potential exposure of patients or users to the substance,

(b) an analysis of possible alternative substances, materials or designs, including, where available, information on independent research, peer-reviewed studies, scientific opinions of relevant scientific committees and an analysis of the availability of these alternatives,

(c) a reason why possible substitutes of substances and/or materials, if available, or changes in design, if feasible, are not appropriate in relation to maintaining the functionality, performance and benefit/risk ratio of the product, taking into account whether the intended use of these products includes the treatment of children or pregnant or breastfeeding women or other patient groups considered particularly vulnerable to these substances and/or materials; and

(d) where applicable and available, the latest relevant scientific committee guidelines in accordance with Sections 10.4.3. and 10.4.4.

COM has been required first to have a guideline on phthalates drawn up through the Scientific Committee, which is already accomplished[242], and then Commission Guidelines on other substances, as necessary.
The presence of these substances shall be indicated in the form of a list in the **labelling** of the MD. If the treatment of vulnerable groups (children, pregnant women, nursing and other vulnerable groups) is also planned, the **instructions for use** must contain information on residual risks and, if necessary, appropriate precautions for these patient groups.

---

[241] Regulation (EU) No 528/2012 of the European Parliament and the Council of 22 May 2012 concerning the making available on the market of and use of biocidal products (OJ L 167, 27.6.2012, p. 1).
[242] https://ec.europa.eu/health/document/download/831f9b60-88de-4197-858f-d001c5b0cc26_en

Fig. 18 IVDR: Annex I Overview

IVDR Annex I

I. General requirements

Performance Evaluation	Risk-Management

II. Requirements regarding Performance, Design and Manufacture

9. Performance Characteristics
a) analytical performance
b) clinical performance
10. Chemical, physical and biological properties
11. Infection and microbial contamination
12. Materials of biological origin
13. Construction, interaction with environment
14. Measuring function
15. Protection against Radiation
16. Electronic programmable systems, Software
17. IVD with energy source
18. Mechanical and thermal risks
19. Risks by lay-use or near-patient testing

III. Information supplied with IVD

20.1. General information Requirements
20.2. Information on label
20.3. Sterile packaging
20.4. Instructions for use

5.5. Important changes[243] to the General Safety and Performance Requirements for IVDs in Annex I

See overview in Fig. 18.

Chapter I (General requirements) of Annex I centers on **performance evaluation** (see chapter VII in this book) and the **risk management system[244]**.

Chap. II and Chap. III of Annex I of the IVDR contain more specific aspects of risk management and performance:

IVDR: Annex I, Chapter II: Requirements regarding Performance, Design and Manufacture

Section 9: Performance Characteristics

Here the important parameters for **analytical performance** and **clinical (diagnostic) performance**, which are to be worked off within the scope of the performance evaluation, are explicitly listed (see Tab. 16). These are largely unchanged from the IVD Directive and have central importance in the IVD regulatory system; the definitions for many of these parameters can now be found in Art. 2 of the IVDR.

These performances (to be assured over the life-cycle of the IVD) will have to be evaluated, if applicable, also in specific application scenarios, such as for IVD for self-testing and IVD for near-patient testing.

The metrological traceability of calibrators and calibration materials must be ensured.

Section 10: Chemical, physical and biological properties

This section is significantly slimmer in the IVDR than the corresponding one in MDR due to the lack of invasive body contact of the IVDs. The primary objective here is the elimination/minimization of impairments of the analytical performance by possible physical and/or chemical interferences, as far as the intended purpose of the IVD permits. The exposure to released pollutants, including residues, must be minimised; with regard to the avoidance

---

[243] Compared to the previous Directive!
[244] See chapter 5.1. in this book

of hazards from CMR substances and substances with endocrine activity (endocrine disruptors - ED), there are simplified provisions compared to MDR.

Section 11: Infection and microbial contamination

Widely like the corresponding section in the MDR.

IVDs and their manufacture must be designed in such a way that the risk of infection for users and possibly other persons is excluded or, if this is not possible, kept as low as possible. Particular attention must be paid to easy and safe handling by design. Microbial leakage from the device and/or microbial exposure during use and the risk of microbial contamination of the device (or in case of specimen receptacles, the risk of contamination of the specimen) should be reduced as far as possible. Section 11.3. now explicitly refers to **validated sterilization procedures**[245].

Section 12: Products incorporating materials of biological origin

Where the products contain tissues, cells and substances of animal, human or microbial origin, the selection of sources, processing, preservation, testing and treatment of such tissues, cells and substances and the control procedures shall be carried out in such a way as to ensure safety for users or third parties.

In particular, recognized validated processes for elimination or inactivation during the manufacturing process shall ensure protection against microbial and other transmissible pathogens. This may not apply to certain products if the activity of the microbial agent or other transmissible agent is part of the intended use of the product or if such an elimination or inactivation process would impair the performance of the product.

....

Section 13: Construction of devices and interaction with their environment

If the device is intended for use in combination with other devices or equipment, the whole combination, including the connection system, shall be

---

[245] If applicable; see wealth of relevant harmonised standards in chapter 1.4.4 of this book.

safe and shall not impair the specified performances of the devices. Any restrictions on use applying to such combinations shall be indicated on the label and/or in the instructions for use.

Devices shall be designed and manufactured in such a way as to remove or reduce as far as possible:

- Risks of injury,
- risks connected with reasonably foreseeable external influences or environmental conditions, such as magnetic fields, external electrical and electromagnetic effects, ...
- risks through contacts with materials, liquids, substances, ...
- the risks associated with the possible negative interaction between software and the IT environment within which it operates and interacts;
- risks of accidental ingress of substances, ...
- risk of incorrect identification of specimens and the risk of erroneous results, ...
- risks of any foreseeable interference with other devices.

Devices shall be designed and manufactured in such a way as to minimise the risks of fire or explosion, ...

Devices shall be designed and manufactured in such a way that adjustment, calibration, and maintenance can be done safely and effectively;

Devices that are intended to be operated together with other devices or products shall be designed and manufactured in such a way that the interoperability and compatibility are reliable and safe.

Devices shall be designed and manufactured in such a way as to facilitate their safe disposal and the safe disposal of related waste substances by users, or other person, ...

The measuring, monitoring or display scale (including colour change and other visual indicators) shall be designed and manufactured in line with ergonomic principles, ...

Section 16: Electronic Programmable Systems - Devices that incorporate electronic programmable systems and Software that are devices in themselves[246]

The requirements are identical to those in section 17 of Annex I of MDR. There has been a significant expansion and deepening of the requirements here:

16.1 Products that include electronic programmable systems, including software, or software that are devices in themselves, shall be designed to **ensure repeatability, reliability and performance** in accordance with their intended use. In the event of a single fault condition, appropriate means must be adopted to eliminate or reduce as far as possible consequent risks or impairments of performance.

16.2 For devices that incorporate software or for software that are devices in themselves, the software shall be developed and manufactured in accordance with the state of the art taking into account the **principles of development life cycle[247], risk management, including information security, verification and validation**.

16.3 Software referred to in this Section that is intended to be used in combination with **mobile computing platforms** shall be designed and manufactured taking into account the specific features of the mobile platform (e.g. size and contrast ratio of the screen) and the **external factors related to their use** (varying environment as regards level of light or noise).

16.4. Manufacturers shall set out minimum requirements concerning **hardware, IT networks characteristics and IT security measures, including protection against unauthorised access**, necessary to run the software as intended.

Section 17: Products connected to or equipped with an energy source

The requirements here are largely based on those of the IVD Directive. Devices where the safety of the patient depends on an internal power supply

---

[246] In newer MDCG terminology addressed as Medical Device Software (MDSW), see MDCG 2019.11: Qualification and classification of software - Regulation (EU) 2017/745 and Regulation (EU) 2017/746; in IMDRF terminology now called Software as a MD (SaMD) see www.imdrf.org

[247] See also EN 62304 Medical device software - Software life-cycle processes

shall be equipped with a means of determining the state of the power supply and an appropriate warning or indication for when the capacity of the power supply becomes critical. If necessary, such warning or indication shall be given prior to the power supply becoming critical.

Additions have been made to IVDs with an internal energy source, which now requires not only a means to check the state of power supply, but also a warning or display that is activated before or when the state of charge of the energy source reaches a critical level.

Active and passive immunity against electromagnetic interference with possible impairment of the function of the IVD or other IVDs or other products during normal operation is also required. Accidental electric shocks should be avoided as far as possible both during normal use and in the event of a single fault condition

.

.....

Section 19: Protection against the risks of products intended for self-testing or near-patient testing

In addition to the special requirements for IVDs for self-testing already existing in Directive 98/79/EC, IVDs for near-patent testing (POCT) are now also included under this heading.

19.1. *Devices intended for self-testing or near-patient testing shall be designed and manufactured in such a way that they perform appropriately for their intended purpose taking into account the skills and the means available to the intended user and the influence resulting from variation that can be reasonably anticipated in the intended user's technique and environment. The information and instructions provided by the manufacturer shall be easy for the intended user to understand and apply in order to correctly interpret the result provided by the device and to avoid misleading information. In the case of near-patient testing, the information and the instructions provided by the manufacturer shall make clear the level of training, qualifications and/or experience required by the user.*

19.2. *Devices intended for self-testing or near-patient testing must be designed and manufactured in such a way as to:*

  a) *ensure that the device can be used safely and accurately by the intended user at all stages of the procedure if necessary, after appropriate training and/or information; and*

b) reduce as far as possible the risk of error by the intended user in the handling of the device and, if applicable, the specimen, and also in the interpretation of the results.

19.3. Devices intended for self-testing and near-patient testing must, where feasible, include a procedure by which the intended user:

a) can verify that, at the time of use, the device will perform as intended by the manufacturer; and

b) be warned if the device has failed to provide a valid result.

IVDR: Annex I, Chapter III: Requirements for the information provided with the device

Section 20: Label and Instructions for use

This section is again extremely detailed for a New Approach act.

Section 20.1. deals with the **general conditions for the provision of information in labelling and instructions for use**, which takes account of further developments in this area; the exact identification of IVDs and manufacturers and the information on safety and performance relevant for users, patients and third parties are in the foreground. Electronic instructions for professional use, including POCT, are now also possible.

Human-readable information must always be available but can be supplemented by e.g. RFID or barcodes.

Also note that harmonised symbols and identification colours in harmonised standards and common specifications, where available, are binding. Hazard pictograms and labelling requirements according to Regulation (EC) 1272/2008[248] and the safety data sheet according to Regulation (EU) No. 1907/2006[249] must also be observed (if information is not completely contained in the instructions for use).

You should work through Sections 20.2 (Labelling), 20.3. (Sterile packaging) and 20.4 (Instructions for Use) in a meticulous checklist-like manner when designing the respective labels and instructions for use, where applicable in individual cases. These passages have been elaborated in much more detail than the previous IVD Directive, especially with regard to analytical performance and clinical performance, target groups and areas of application. For

---

[248] REGULATION (EC) No 1272/2008 OF THE EUROPEAN PARLIAMENT AND OF THE COUNCIL of 16 December 2008 on classification, labelling and packaging of substances and mixtures, amending and repealing Directives 67/548/EEC and 1999/45/EC, and amending Regulation (EC) No 1907/2006
[249] REGULATION (EC) No 1907/2006 OF THE EUROPEAN PARLIAMENT AND OF THE COUNCIL of 18 December 2006 concerning the Registration, Evaluation, Authorisation and Restriction of Chemicals (**REACH**), establishing a European Chemicals Agency, amending Directive 1999/45/EC and repealing Council Regulation (EEC) No 793/93 and Commission Regulation (EC) No 1488/94 as well as Council Directive 76/769/EEC and Commission Directives 91/155/EEC, 93/67/EEC, 93/105/EC and 2000/21/EC

IVD for self-testing, POCT or sterile packaging there are now additional or separate labelling requirements.

See also:
EN ISO 15223-1: Medical devices — Symbols to be used with medical device labels, labelling and information to be supplied — Part 1: General requirements (harmonised European symbols and identification colors will be binding!);
EN ISO 20417 Medical devices — Information to be supplied by the manufacturer; and labelling and/or IFU-elements in specific product (group) standards.
EN ISO 18113-series: In vitro diagnostic medical devices - Information supplied by the manufacturer (labelling)
You may also find additional hints on labelling and IFU in more product specific standards

Another piece of information to be provided for IVDs of classes C+D is the **Summary on Safety and Performance** (SSP) according to Art. 29 (see chapter VII Performance Evaluation in this book)

Chapter 6. Clinical evaluation of medical devices

MDR: Art. 2 (44); Art. 61 and Annex XIV

> *"clinical evaluation" means a systematic and planned process to continuously generate, collect, analyse and assess the clinical data pertaining to a device in order to verify the safety and performance, including clinical benefits, of the device when used as intended by the manufacturer;*

MDR places great emphasis on clinical evaluation as an **active, systematic life cycle process based on a clinical evaluation plan and leading to a clinical evaluation report, to be contiuously updated by PMCF[250]**; the clinical evaluation must be carried out by the manufacturer under his QMS.

Sources:
Legal text:
MDR: Art. 2 definitions; Art. 61 and Annex XIV
Guidance:
Still most important and useful: **MEDDEV 2.7.1 rev. 4**[251]: Clinical evaluation: Guide for manufacturers and notified bodies; developed under the Directives MDD and AIMDD, version 2007/47/EC, still the most important and useful guidance also under the MDR; MDR has taken strong bonds from guideline MEDDEV 2.7.1 rev.4 on Clinical Evaluation, developed in parallel with MDR.
MDCG Guidance[252]:
MDCG 2020-13 Clinical evaluation assessment report template
MDCG 2020-8   Guidance on PMCF evaluation report template
MDCG 2020-7   Guidance on PMCF plan template
MDCG 2020-6   Guidance on sufficient clinical evidence for legacy devices
MDCG 2020-5   Guidance on clinical evaluation – Equivalence
MDCG 2020-1   Guidance on clinical evaluation (MDR) / Performance eval-uation (IVDR) of medical device software
MDCG 2019-9   Summary of safety and clinical performance
MDCG Guidancies on clinical investigation may also be helpful.
IMDRF Guidelines:
IMDRF MDCE WG/N56FINAL: 2019 Clinical Evaluation

---

[250] PMCF: Post Market Clinical Follow-up
[251] https://ec.europa.eu/docsroom/documents/17522/attachments/1/translations/
[252] https://ec.europa.eu/health/md_sector/new_regulations/guidance_en

Other Guidance or Sources:

Documents, to be elaborated under the EU Horizon 2020 project CORE MD (Coordinating Research and Evidence for Medical Devices; Improved methods for clinical investigation and evaluation of high-risk medical devices): https://www.core-md.eu/ ;

Clinical evidence guidelines: Medical devices, of the Australian Competent Authority TGA (Version Nov. 2021): https://www.tga.gov.au/resource/clinical-evidence-guidelines-medical-devices

Guidance developed by (European or other reliable) specialist clinical societies, like European Cardiological SOCIETY; Orthopedic societies like EFFORT or EARN (European Arthroplasty Register Network); and many others;

HTA-reports[253], EbM systematic reviews may also provide helpful input.

(Harmonized) European and international standards, which contain more and more useful hints for clinical evaluation and investigation of specific medical devices.

The clinical evaluation is part of the proof of compliance with the general safety and performance requirements according to Annex I, see also Tab. 10.

Tab. 10 MDR: Aspects to be Covered by Clinical Evaluation in Annex I.I.

The following aspects of Annex I.I. address in particular aspects to be demonstrated by clinical evaluation:
▪ MDs provide the intended performance and are suitable for achieving the intended purpose;
▪ Safety and effectiveness;
▪ no compromising of clinical condition, safety and health;
▪ positive benefit/risk ratio;
▪ compatible with a high degree of health protection and safety;
▪ State of the art;
▪ Acceptability of minimized! residual risks and side effects related to clinical performance and clinical benefits of MD;
• These points and the aspects required in Art. 61 and Annex XIV must be processed within the framework of the clinical evaluation.

---

[253] Health technology assessment; EbM Evidence based Medicine, e.g. those of EUnetHTA https://www.eunethta.eu/ and its principles or Cochrane reports https://www.cochrane.org/

If necessary, certain points of Chapter II of Annex I (e.g. the added value of ancillary pharmaceuticals or non-viable components of human, animal or organismic origin, the clinical evaluation of medical device software (MDSW)[254] or usability aspects, specifically in MD for self-use) are relevant in the context of clinical evaluation; Chapter III of Annex I now contains more clinical information in the labelling and instructions for use, which must also be underpinned by the clinical evaluation.

The **specification of the clinical benefit/risk determination** is now a key issue of clinical evaluation. Both clinical benefits and clinical safety (incl. clinical risks and undesirable side effects) have to be specified qualitatively and as far as possible quantitatively[255] with regard to:

- Type of effect;
- strength, Intensity, extent of effects;
- Duration of effects and
- Frequency/probability of effects in the target group(s) defined as precisely as possible by indications and contraindications

(see Tab. 11[256]).

---

[254] See also MDCG 2020-1: Guidance on clinical evaluation (MDR) / Performance evaluation (IVDR) of medical device software

[255] MEDDEV 2.7.1. rev 4 concedes, that for some well-established technologies of low risk, qualitative assessment may be all that is reasonably possible; this has to be justified in any case. A guidance is in preparation (see roadmap of CAMD)

[256] See also various guidance by FDA/CDRH on benefit-risk determination

Tab. 11 Clinical Specification of Benefit/Risk-Determination

Clinical Specification of Benefit/Risk-Determination acc to MDR and MEDDEV 2.7.1. rev 4		
Qualitative/Quantitative determination, differentiated for:		
Clinical Benefits	Type of effects	Clinical safety (incl. clinical risks and unde- sireable side- effects)
	Strength, intensity, extent	
	Duration	
	Frequency/Probability in defined target group(s)/Indi- cations	

The following terms now play an important role in clinical evaluation in MDR[257]:

Tab. 12 Clinical Evaluation of MD: Important Definitions in MDR

'clinical data' means information concerning safety or performance that is gener- ated from the use of a device and is sourced from the following: — clinical investigation(s) of the device concerned, — clinical investigation(s) or other studies reported in scientific literature, of a de- vice for which equivalence to the device in question can be demonstrated, — reports published in peer reviewed scientific literature on other clinical experi- ence of either the device in question or a device for which equivalence to the device in question can be demonstrated, — clinically relevant information coming from post-market surveillance, in particu- lar the post-market clinical follow-up;
'clinical evidence' means clinical data and clinical evaluation results pertaining to a device of a sufficient amount and quality to allow a qualified assessment of whether the device is safe and achieves the intended clinical benefit(s), when used as in- tended by the manufacturer;
'clinical performance' means the ability of a device, resulting from any direct or in- direct medical effects which stem from its technical or functional characteristics, in- cluding diagnostic characteristics, to achieve its intended purpose as claimed by the manufacturer, thereby leading to a clinical benefit for patients, when used as in- tended by the manufacturer;

---

[257] MDR: Art. 2 (48), (51)-(53)

*'**clinical benefit**' means the positive impact of a device on the health of an individual, expressed in terms of a meaningful, measurable, patient-relevant clinical outcome(s), including outcome(s) related to diagnosis, or a positive impact on patient management or public health;*

Fig. 19 MDR: Steps to Clinical Evaluation

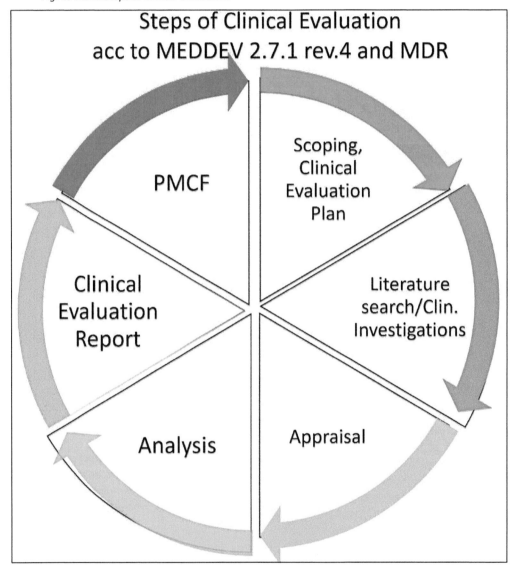

Steps of Clinical Evaluation acc to MEDDEV 2.7.1 rev.4 and MDR

PMCF

Scoping, Clinical Evaluation Plan

Clinical Evaluation Report

Literature search/Clin. Investigations

Analysis

Appraisal

Another important issue of clinical evaluation, taken over from MEDDEV 2.7.1. rev 4[258], is a **defined step/stage approach of clinical evaluation** in the MDR (see Fig. 19):

Step 0: Scoping and clinical evaluation plan
(incl. clinical development plan and PMCF plan);

Scoping defines the framework for clinical evaluation with focus on a clear description of the device and it's intended purpose/use, including planned variants, all necessary accessories and intended product combinations, as well as alleged equivalences[259] with another MD (the predicate device). On the basis of this scoping, the **clinical evaluation plan**[260], including a **clinical development plan** and a post-market clinical follow-up plan (**PMCF plan**) can be established. The clinical evaluation plan involves the specification of pa-tient-relevant measurable outcomes for clinical benefit, efficacy/effective-ness, clinical performance and for clinical safety (including [residual] clinical risks and undesireable side effects) and the precise definitions of indications and contraindications as well as of target groups[261] as the core elements.

---

[258] And originating largely from the GHTF/IMDRF Guideline http://www.im-drf.org/docs/ghtf/final/sg5/technical-docs/ghtf-sg5-n2r8-2007-clinical-evaluation-070501.pdf : Guideline on Clinical Evaluation

[259] Please note that for a claimed predicate device to be equivalent, **technical, biological and clinical equivalence and relevant data access** (including for the clinical data) must be given, see MDR: Annex XIV.A.3 and MDCG 2020-5: Guidance on clinical evaluation – Equivalence

[260] See details in MDR: Annex XIV.A.1.a)

[261] Search for relevant and meaningful outcomes and how to measure them may be found in international data banks of clinical trials, like www.clinicaltrials.gov or ICTRP of WHO http://apps.who.int/trialsearch/ or systematic reviews or HTA- and EbM- assessments. See http://onlinelibrary.wiley.com/cochranelibrary/search?searchRow.searchOptions.search-Products=clinicalTrialsDoi (Cochrane library) and https://www.crd.york.ac.uk/CRDWeb/ Center for Reviews and Dissemination of the University of York.
https://www.eunethta.eu/European network for HTA
http://eprints.hta.lbg.ac.at/view/types/dsd.html Decision Support Documents of the Lud-wig-Boltzmann Institute for HTA in Austria with a lot of HTA assessments for medical devices with literature search according to the PICO-scheme.
https://www.iqwig.de/de/projekte-ergebnisse/publikationen/iqwig-berichte.1071.html Pro-ject reports by the German IQWIG, with a lot of HTA assessments of medical devices and lit-erature search according to the PICO-scheme.

These are the prerequisites necessary for literature search, clinical investigations' set-up, PMCF and comparison with the state of the art[262].

Please note, that for Medical Device Software (MDSW), MDCG 2020-1 has provided a specific non-legally binding guidance document on clinical evaluation following the rationale of performance evaluation of IVDs[263]; this guidance has been inspired by the corresponding IMDRF-guidance.

Step 1: Identification and generation of relevant clinical data

especially through literature search(es) and clinical investigation(s) as well as other sources of valid clinical data[264], e.g. PMCF-data;

the literature searches[265] concern

- the **Medical Device itself** in its intended conditions of application and
- the determination of the recognized **state of the art** in the medical field of application[266].

Specifically remarkable also: http://www.comet-initiative.org/ (Core Outcome Measures in Effectiveness Trials) with database and search function. This will be useful for designing clinical investigations or for literature search and to ease benchmarking with the state of the art in the relevant medical field.

[262] See MDR: Annex I.I.1. and Art. 61(3) c)

[263] MDCG 2020-1: Guidance on clinical evaluation (MDR) / Performance evaluation (IVDR) of medical device software; please note, that contrary to MDSW, **software that is intended to drive or influence a medical device**, for which the manufacturer does not claim any medical intended purpose, the CLINICAL EVIDENCE is provided within the context of the driven or influenced device and is therefore out of the scope of this MDCG-document. See as a precursor of this MDCG guidance the related IMDRF guidance: http://www.imdrf.org/docs/imdrf/final/technical/imdrf-tech-170921-samd-n41-clinical-evaluation_1.pdf

[264] See definition of 'clinical data' indicating the possible routes of generating relevant clinical data, which have to be taken into account in this step.

[265] A possible help for the Literature Search Report and the methods behind can be found in the GHTF/IMDRF Guidance „Clinical Evaluation", Appendix B: A Possible Format for the Literature Search Report and Appendix C: A possible methodology for documenting the screening and selection of literature within a literature search report http://www.imdrf.org/docs/imdrf/final/technical/imdrf-tech-191010-mdce-n56.pdf

A deeper instruction for proper scientific literature search for MD can be found in: Ecker, Labek, et.al.: Clinical Evaluation and Investigation of Medical Devices under the new EU-Regulation; BoD Books on Demand, Norderstedt, Germany, 2020.

[266] Often provided by Evidence based Medicine reviews, Cochrane Reports; HTA-Assessments, see http://apps.who.int/iris/bitstream/handle/10665/44564/9789241501361_eng.pdf;jsessionid=A3939AE214141D5476A58F3FE1E6FABE?sequence=1 ;

The **Literature Search Protocol** describes the planning of the literature search(es) with objectives and methodology for the WHAT, WHERE and HOW of the search. The **literature search report**[267] describes the performance of the search, the loyalty to the plan, with justification for deviations, and the results of the literature search. The **full texts** of the relevant literature references found are attached to the Clinical Evaluation Report.

For clinical investigations, see chapter VIII of this book. Clinical investigations will - under the MDR - be obligatory for implantable MDs and Class III MDs, with some exemptions, see MDR: Art. 61 (4)-(7). For PMCF see step 5 below.

Step 2: Appraisal (assessment and weighting of available clinical data);
The clinical data (manufacturer's own clinical investigations and other clinical data he has access to (e.g. see Art. 61, also his PMCF data) and those from the literature search(es)) established in step 1 must now be evaluated according to the following criteria:

- **Relevance** for the qualitative and/or quantitative determination of the clinical benefit/risk-safety profile of the MD (or MD shown as equivalent) in the intended application areas (incl. target groups, indications, contraindications, etc.) (see Tab. 11);
- Relevance for determining the **current state of the art** in the intended medical field of application for assessing the acceptability of the clinical benefit/risk profile of your MD[268];
- Assessment of the **methodological and scientific quality** of the individual clinical data (sensitivity of the reported outcomes to confounders, bias, random error, dubious and multiple reporting, etc.;

---

https://www.eunethta.eu/ ; https://www.cochrane.org/ ;
Important national HTA institutes in device area: e.g. https://hta.lbg.ac.at/page/homepage/en ; https://www.iqwig.de/en/home.2724.html ; https://www.nice.org.uk/ ;
[267] See here GHTF/IMDRF Guidance „Clinical Evaluation", Appendix B: A Possible Format for the Literature Search Report and Appendix C: A possible methodology for documenting the screening and selection of literature within a literature search report: http://www.imdrf.org/docs/imdrf/final/technical/imdrf-tech-191010-mdce-n56.pdf
[268] See MDR: Annex I.I.1. and Art. 61(3) c) where currently available alternative treatment options for that purpose have to be considered in the clinical evaluation

- How are the individual clinical data to be **weight** for their contribution to generate clinical evidence for clinical safety and efficacy/effectiveness based on this appraisal[269]?

Maximum weight is usually achieved in well-run randomised, controlled clinical trials (**RCTs**). The MEDDEV 2.7.1 rev 4 concludes that RCTs are not always practical and that other study designs may be acceptable[270]. It is also pointed out in particular that for well-established low-risk technologies[271], qualitative rather than quantitative appraisals can often be acceptable, but this has to be justified in any case.

Stage 3: Analysis: the next task is a structured analysis of the weighted clinical data and drawing conclusions with regard to compliance with applicable General Safety and Performance Requirements of Annex I. The main issues here are: safety and effectiveness; positive clinical benefit/risk ratio (Tab. 10), which is acceptable against the state of the art in the intended areas of medical application (target groups, indications with consideration of contraindications); high level of health protection etc (see Tab. 11). Another important analysis concerns gaps in clinical evidence that will have to be closed by targeted clinical investigations or specific PMCF activities. According to the MEDDEV, special considerations can apply to "well established technologies (of low risk)", devices for unmet medical needs and breakthrough products[272]. If necessary, the "added value" of ancillary pharmaceutical components or of ancillary non-viable tissues, cells, derivatives of animal or human origin[273] or lay usability or for clinical evaluation of Medical Device Software (MDSW) must also be documented by clinical data and taken into account in the analysis.

Other tasks in the analysis step are:

---

[269] See e.g. GHTF/IMDRF: http://www.imdrf.org/docs/imdrf/final/technical/imdrf-tech-191010-mdce-n56.pdf: Guideline on Clinical Evaluation, Appendix F: A Possible Method of Appraisal

[270] See e.g. GHTF/IMDRF: http://www.imdrf.org/docs/imdrf/final/technical/imdrf-tech-191010-mdce-n56.pdf Guideline on Clinical Evaluation, Appendix E: Some Examples to Assist with the Formulation of Criteria

[271] acc to CAMD roadmap, a guideline is in preparation on well-established technologies

[272] The roadmap of the CAMD contains indications of planned guidance for those specific issues

[273] non-viable derivatives of human origin in principal function are theoretically possible, see Art. 1.6.g), 2nd half-sentence

- the examination of the planned **Summary of Safety and Clinical Performance (SSCP)** according to Art. 32 of the MDR (for Class III and implantable devices)[274] and
- examination of planned **implant information** according to Art. 18[275].
- Don't forget the clinical information to be provided in **labelling** and **instructions for use** and in **advertising materials**,
- the documentation for custom-made devices[276] and the
- entries in the technical documentation (MDR: Annex II.6, especially the CER and its updates and annexed documents, see Tab. 13!).

Stage 4: Preparation and updating of the Clinical Evaluation Report (CER) as the most important summary document of the clinical evaluation and essential part of the technical documentation. The CER documents the clinical evaluation process with its stages and results and constitutes the clinical evidence for MDs and compliance with the clinically relevant GSPR. A possible structure and possible associated contents of the CER are shown in Tab. 13. Don't forget annexing the associated materials for clinical evaluation, in particular for clinical investigations or literature search and its results (in full text), which is strongly recommended with regard to the NB's time and work economy when assessing the clinical evaluation[277].

Stage 5: Post-market clinical follow-up (PMCF; MDR: Annex XIV.B). PMCF is based on a **PMCF plan**[278], **general**[279] and **specific PMCF methods** and the **PMCF evaluation reports**[280], which serve to update clinical evaluation, PMS and risk management. PMCF includes, for example, long-term studies[281] and

---

[274] See MDCG 2019-9: Summary of safety and clinical performance

[275] MDCG 2019-8 v2: Guidance document implant card on the application of Article 18 Regulation (EU) 2017/745 on medical devices

[276] See MDR: Annex XIII.2

[277] See specifically in MEDDEV 2.7.1 rev 4: Appendices A9-11; Checklist in Appendix A10; see also: validation checklist of the NB TUEV SUED under: http://www.tuev-sued.de/uploads/images/1468322106100422581021/tuev-sued-validation-checklist-of-clinical-evidence-en.pdf

[278] See here MDCG 2020-7: Guidance on PMCF plan template

[279] There are initial considerations on how to use (valid) BIG DATA in that.

[280] See here MDCG 2020-8: Guidance on PMCF evaluation report template

[281] E.g. in coronary stents it is current practice to consent patients for 5 years for clinical investigations, where pivotal results after 2y may be presented for initial conformity assessment and the following 3 years would serve for additional PMCF study data.

implant register[282] evaluations. The update via PMCF evaluation reports must be carried out at least once a year for implants and Class III-MDs.

Tab. 13 MDR: Possible Structure and Content of CER

Possible structure	Possible content acc to MDR and MEDDEV
1.Executive summary	Concise description of MD, it's mode of action, it's intended purpose/use and indication(s), summary of the steps of clinical evaluation performed and their results, summary of clinical evidence gathered, esp. for clinical benefit/risk determination in the intended target group(s) and indication(s), proof of acceptability of benefit/risk profile against the state of the art in the resp. medical field, poss. with gap analysis.
2.Scope and clinical evaluation plan	See specifically MDR: Annex XIV.A.1.a) with detailed checklist
3. clin. background; current state of knowledge; state of the art in the resp. medical field(s)	See specifically Appendix A8 of MEDDEV 2.7.1 rev 4; results of literature search report concerning the state of the art and alternative treatment options in the resp. medical field(s)
4. search and generation of pertinent clinical data	
a) sources of clinical data; route(s) chosen	Justification of route(s) chosen or excluded concerning definition of "clinical data" in MDR: Art. 2 (48): <ul><li>clinical investigation(s) of the device concerned,</li><li>clinical investigation(s) or other studies reported in scientific literature, of a device for</li></ul>

	which equivalence to the device in question can be demonstrated, • reports published in peer reviewed scientific literature on other clinical experience of either the device in question or a device for which equivalence to the device in question can be demonstrated, • clinically relevant information coming from post-market surveillance, in particular the PMCF;
b) demonstration of equivalence, if used	Please note the required technical, biological **and** clinical equivalence[283] **and** data access!
c) own clinical data of manufacturer	Clinical development plan and Clinical Investigation Reports, Summaries and publications of corresponding exploratory and confirmatory clinical investigation(s) and PMCF-studies and other relevant clinical PMCF/PMS-data; evidence of conformity of clinical investigations with requirements of Chapter VI and Annex XV of MDR and with EN ISO 14155
d) Literature search	Literature search protocol(s) and literature search report(s) and annexed full texts of relevant literature
e) Appraisal	Appraisal-plan; results of check for relevance to MD and application; results of check for methodological-scientific quality of clinical data; weighting of results; Appraisal-report
f) Analysis	Analysis-Plan and -Report; Gap-analysis; specific considerations concerning, if applicable, well established technologies of low risk, breakthrough devices and unmet medical needs;
5. Conclusions	Conclusions, mainly as a result of step 3, concerning:

---

[283] For details see specifically MDR: Annex XIV.A.3; MDCG 2020-5: Guidance on clinical evaluation – Equivalence

	o meeting the General Safety and Performance Requirements set out in Annex I which apply to the MD, and its intended purpose and use, to be demonstrated with clinical data;
	o the clinical benefit(s), clinical performance(s), effectiveness, based on patient-relevant, measurable outcomes;
	o the clinical safety of the MD based on relevant parameters, incl. to clinically relevant rest-risks and unintended side-effects;
	o the intended medical fields of application, incl. exactly defined target groups, indications, contraindications;
	o the benefit/risk determination and the acceptability of the benefit/risk ratio of the MD against the state of the art in the intended medical field, based on relevant outcomes for clinical safety and efficacy/effectiveness;
	o the benefit/risk ratio under specific consideration of unintended side-effects;
	o the consistency of the claims, statements, documents and advertising of the manufacturer on the safety, effectiveness, benefit/risk determination, acceptability of benefit/risk ratio towards the results of the clinical evaluation;
	o the results of the gap analysis with conclusions on unresolved issues and unanswered questions;
	o conclusions to the need of further clinical investigation(s) and/or necessary PMCF activities;
6a. PMCF	See MDR: Annex XIV.B: this goes beyond the MEDDEV and is legally binding:

168

	PMCF-Plan[284]; results of general and specific PMCF methods; PMCF-Evaluation Reports[285] and conclusions for adaptation of clinical evaluation;
6b. Date of next update of clinical evaluation, with justification	MDR: Art. 61 (11) requires at least yearly update of the PMCF Evaluation Report for implants and Class III MDs; the MEDDEV required at least a yearly update for significant risk MDs or if the MD is not based on a well-established technology. For other MDs an interval of 2-5 years is recommended, with a justification and in line with the NB.
7. Date and Signature(s)	Date and version of the CER; Statement of the clinical evaluator(s), that he/she/they agree(s) with the CER; date(s), name(s) and signature(s) of the evaluator(s); Final release of the CER by the manufacturer: date, name and signature
8. Qualifications of the clinical evaluator(s)	See section 6.4. of the MEDDEV, incl. Declaration(s) of Interest[286]
9. References:	In principle, all clinical data, results and conclusions should be clearly referenced to appropriate sources, literature references or documents etc.
10. Annexed Documents (important for timely assessment by NB[287]!)	If applicable and not already included in the CER, e.g. Clinical Evaluation Plan; Clinical Development Plan; PMCF-Plan; Literature-Search-Protocol(s) and Literature-Search-Re-

---

[284] See template in MDCG 2020-7
[285] See template in MDCG 2020-8
[286] See MEDDEV 2.7.1. rev. 4: Section 6.4. and App. A11 (Declaration of Interest DoI)
[287] The NB has to issue a **Clinical Evaluation Assessment Report – CEAR,** see MDCG 2020-13: 'Clinical evaluation assessment report template' to see what the NB will have to look at during clinical evaluation assessment; see MDR: Annex IX.II.4.8; missing documents will delay assessment by NB

	ports as well as full texts of relevant publication(s); Appraisal-Plan; Appraisal-Report; Analysis-Plan; Analysis-Report; To the clinical investigation(s) of the manufacturer:[288] and PMCF-Studies: Clinical Investigation Reports, Summaries und Publication(s); additional documents (of CAs and ethics committee(s); CIP and IB); PMCF Evaluation Reports; all justifications for the lack of clinical investigations acc. to MDR: Art. 61 (6)-(8); (draft) Summary on Safety and Clinical Performance (SSCP)[289]; label and IFU; Device History; details to the clinical. evaluator(s)[290], incl. DoI;

Considerations concerning specific clinical evaluations

1) Clinical evaluation of Medical Device Software (MDSW)

A special feature is the clinical evaluation of Medical Device Software (MDSW[291]) with its often diagnostic, predictive and prognostic functions. Corresponding preliminary work has been done by the IMDRF with the guideline "Software as a Medical Device (SaMD) Clinical Evaluation". MDCG 2020-1 follows partly this global guideline; but it also remains responsive to the step-by-step approach of clinical evaluation outlined in MEDDEV 2.7.1 rev.4, with the sequence of Clinical Evaluation Plan, identification of relevant clinical data (through literature review, clinical investigations and other sources of valid clinical data, including PMCF data), assessment and analysis of these data, the Clinical Evaluation Report and subsequent PMCF for updates.

---

[288] If applicable also to clinical investigations to which the manufacturer has access to acc. to MDR: Art. 61 (5).

[289] The draft SSCP has acc. to MDR: Art. 32 to be validated by the NB and then uploaded to EUDAMED; see also MDCG 2019-9: Summary of safety and clinical performance.

[290] see MEDDEV 2.7.1. rev. 4: Section 6.4. and App. A11 (Declaration of Interest DoI)

[291] See MDCG 2020-1: Guidance on clinical evaluation (MDR) / Performance evaluation (IVDR) of medical device software

The scientific methodology, just like it's IMDRF predecessor cited above, follows the concept of performance evaluation for IVDs with the important components:
- Valid clinical association/scientific validity.
- Analytical/technical performance, and
- Clinical performance

Valid clinical association/scientific validity would provide the (scientific) rationale why a particular output (based on defined inputs and algorithms of the MDSW) would serve a particular clinical benefit in relation to particular (patho)physiological clinical conditions, processes or states. Usually this is based on basic research as a starting point and possibly on preliminary results of (mainly) exploratory clinical investigations, expert opinions of medical societies, scientific literature reviews and possibly other valid sources. Usually, scientific validity in the early stages often starts as an indication of a qualitative relationship between the output and the targeted clinical outcome(s) and is further refined step by step, especially through the clinical validation phase, to a semi-quantitative or quantitative correlation.

The **analytical/technical performance** will have to address 2 main issues:
1) Demonstrate the ability of the MDSW to accurately, reliably, reproducibly and precisely generate the intended output from the input data;
2) the MDSW reliably, accurately and consistently fulfils the intended purpose in real-world use under the conditions of usability, IT safety and IT security in the contexts of the intended use environments and the intended users and target groups.
Under point 1), important parameters of analytical performance will be those also used in the IVDR: Annex I.II.9.1.a: analytical sensitivity and specificity, accuracy (from trueness and precision), limits of detection and quantification, linearity, cut-off values, measurement range (interval). Under point 2), parameters such as fitness for purpose in the intended use scenarios, generalisability, availability, confidentiality, integrity, reliability, absence of cybersecurity vulnerabilities would apply.

Clinical performance must demonstrate that users can consistently achieve clinically relevant benefits from the outcomes of MDSWs, based on predictable and reliable use of MDSWs in the intended target populations, operating

171

conditions and conditions of use, including indications, contraindications, well-defined target populations, limitations and warnings.

Clinical performance must be specified according to the parameters, some of which are again specified in the IVDR: Annex I.II.1.b) for clinical performance: Clinical/diagnostic sensitivity and specificity, positive and negative predictive value, positive and negative likelihood ratio, odds ratio, confidence intervals, NNT[292], NNH[293]; complemented by usability aspects .

Please note that for the clinical evaluation of Class III software products, clinical investigations may be legally required under the conditions of the MDR: Art. 64 (4)ff.

2) Well Established Technologies of low risk (WET):

Especially in the case of well-established (proven) technologies of low risk (WET) the identified relevant safety and performance parameters of the medical device will initially, as far as possible, be elaborated with the help of presumptions of conformity from Harmonised Standards (HN) or state-of-the-art standards (SOTAN, eg of ISO or IEC) and Common Specifications (GS) as part of the technical and preclinical evaluation.

Then it must be clarified, what is additionally required beyond technical and preclinical evaluation in terms of clinical safety (incl. undesirable side effects) and clinical performance, clinical effectiveness and clinical benefit.

It must be clarified to what extent the safety and performance parameters of the HN, SOTAN or GS may already completely serve as validated surrogate endpoints for the patient related measurable outcomes for clinical performance and safety as required by the clinical evaluation plan.

On the basis of a reliable PMS system (incl. PMCF) under the MDR, the manufacturer must further ensure that the products based on this established technology can still be considered state of the art in the intended applications and do not have any novelties and that previous experience on the market of this or similar products has shown in particular no new risks or the emergence of superior alternatives, or even medical obsolescence[294].

---

[292] NNT: number needed to treat

[293] NNH: number needed to harm

[294] E.g. a lot of (harmonized) standards for uncomplicated administration of pharmaceuticals (e.g. administration sets, transfer sets, blood administration sets, syringes, needles, tracheal tubes etc) and related biocompatibility standards could serve that purpose.

However, for implants and class III medical devices, the MDR generally requires clinical investigations, with few and highly specified exemptions [see MDR: Art. 61 (4)-(8)]. Post-market clinical follow-up and PMS must in any case be pursued reliably according to Annex XIV.B and Chapter VII.1 and Annex III of MDR.

3) Devices for unmet medical needs and breakthrough devices

Breakthrough devices and devices targeting an 'unmet medical need' are deemed to offer previously unseen major benefits as a result of their early benefit/risk-determination. These may justify higher levels of uncertainty of the clinical benefit/risk-determination for initial conformity assessment. MEDDEV 2.7/1 rev 4, Appendix A8 provides further information on that subject. MDR however has clear provisions for class III and implantable devices as regards the necessity of clinical investigations in Art. 61 (4)-(8).

Higher levels of disclosure of uncertainties on benefits and risks to patients, (lack of) alternatives and gaps in clinical evidence will have to be assured. And the NB has to join in explicitly in its clinical evaluation assessment report (CEAR).

User information in IFU have to refer more in detail, particularly concerning risks, intended purpose and target groups and uncertainties of benefit/risk-determination.

A stringent PMCF-Plan with milestones has to be executed and monitored closely by Notified Bodies. The intended target population has to be limited to the justified area of preliminary positive benefit/risk-determination, where no acceptable alternative is available. To release a breakthrough device from that status requires sufficient clinical evidence on safety and performance/effectiveness accepted by regulatory bodies and Notified Bodies.

4) Use of clinical data of an equivalent medical device

For the constitution of clinical evidence for a medical device, clinical data of a predicate device which is demonstrated to be equivalent to the MD in question can also be used. To demonstrate the equivalence, MDR and the current MEDDEV present almost identical 3 aspects of similarity, which must be fulfilled cumulatively! to prove the equivalence:

Technical: The medical device is of similar design, is used under similar application conditions, has similar specifications and properties including physico-chemical properties such as energy intensity, tensile strength, viscosity, surface finish, wavelength and software algorithms, uses similar development methods where appropriate, and has similar functional principles and critical performance requirements.

Biological: The medical device uses the same materials or substances in contact with the same hu-man tissues or body fluids for a similar type and duration of contact with similar release behaviour of substances, including degradation products and leachables.

Clinical: The medical device is used under the same clinical condition or for the same clinical purpose, including a similar severity and stage of disease, in the same part of the body and in similar patient populations with respect, inter alia, to age, anatomy and physiology, has the same users and performs a similar, authoritative and decisive service with respect to the expected clinical effect for a particular purpose.

These characteristics shall be so uniform that there shall be no clinically significant difference in the safety and clinical performance of the MD claimed to be equivalent, which shall also be adequately scientifically justified.

Manufacturers shall also demonstrate that they have **sufficient access to the (also clinical!) data of the MD** claimed to be similar to demonstrate equivalence on a continuous basis.

With regard to the possible use of clinical investigations of similar MDs, see specifically Art. 61 (4) of the MDR!

See also MDCG 2020-5: Guidance on clinical evaluation – Equivalence

5) Qualification of clinical evaluators

This chapter is not present in the MDR (except for the personnel for clinical investigations, see Art. 62 (6)). Instead however, MEDDEV 2.7.1.rev 4, Section 6.4. explains requirements for the professional qualifications, knowledge and declarations of interest of clinical evaluators (individuals or teams) to ensure an independent and informed clinical evaluation.

The manufacturer must formulate requirements for the clinical evaluators according to the type, purpose, clinical performance and risks of the MD and its intended use and related medical expertise, select its clinical evaluator(s) accordingly and justify the selection in the CER.

The required knowledge and qualifications include:

- <u>General scientific knowledge</u> (research methodology, especially in clinical investigation design and biostatistics); scientific information management and experience in literature search; experience in medical-scientific writing and regulatory background);
- <u>Knowledge of the MD under evaluation and its medical field of application</u> (technology and clinical application; diagnosis and management of clinical application situations; knowledge of medical alternatives and relevant treatment standards; medical specialty)
- <u>Professional qualification, training and experience</u>;
  - relevant academic degree
  - ≥ 5 years documented professional experience
  - ≥ 10 years documented professional experience, if no academic degree is required for the area of application
  - Deviations should be documented and justified.
- The clinical evaluators provide <u>Declarations of Interest (DoI)</u> MEDDEV 2.7.1.rev 4, App. A11, to demonstrate their independence, which describe financial and other interests of the evaluator and close family members relevant to defined time periods that may influence the outcome of the clinical evaluation. Typical contents of the DoI are:

relevant employment, intellectual property or patents, shares, scholarships, grants, participation in clinical investigations or preclinical evaluations, financing of travel and accommodation; lecture fees; etc. The manufacturer should annex the DoIs signed and dated by him and the evaluator to the CER.

Chapter 7. Performance Evaluation of In Vitro Diagnostics

*'**performance evaluation**'[295] means an assessment and analysis of data to establish or verify the scientific validity, the analytical and, where applicable, the clinical performance of a device;*

Sources:

Legal sources:

IVDR: Article 2. (44), (36-41), (49-54); Article 56 and Annex XIII; Annex I.I. and Annex I.II.9.1;

Guidelines:

MDCG 2022-2: Guidance on general principles of clinical evidence for In Vitro Diagnostic medical devices (IVDs)

MDCG 2021-21 Rev.1: Guidance on performance evaluation of SARS-CoV-2 in vitro diagnostic medical devices

MDCG 2020-1: Guidance on clinical evaluation (MDR) / Performance evaluation (IVDR) of medical device software[296]

IMDRF/GHTF: http://www.imdrf.org/documents/doc-ghtf-sg5.asp

(Standards: EN 13612: Performance evaluation of in-vitro diagnostics is based on Directive 98/79/EC and is obsolete; it must first be adapted to IVDR!)

EN ISO 20916, In vitro diagnostic medical devices — Clinical performance studies using specimens from human subjects — Good study practice

The performance evaluation of IVDs is designed by the IVDR as an **active, systematic life cycle process based on a performance evaluation plan, leading to a Performance Evaluation Report (PER), continuously updated by PMPF[297] and to be carried out under the manufacturer's QMS** (Fig. 20).

---

[295] IVDR: Art. 2 (44)

[296] https://ec.europa.eu/health/md_sector/new_regulations/guidance_en

[297] PMPF: Post Market Performance Follow-up

Performance evaluation - here the IVDR follows the concepts of the GHTF/IMDRF - consists of **3 components**[298], which each must be demonstrated in sub-reports and together they constitute the clinical evidence for the IVD in the overall concluding **Performance Evaluation Report (PER):**

Tab. 14 IVDR: 3 Components of Performance Evaluation

- **scientific validity,**
- **analytical performance and**
- **clinical performance**

Tab. 15 Performance Evaluation of IVDs: Important Definitions in IVDR

'scientific validity of an analyte' means the association of an analyte with a clinical condition or a physiological state;
'analytical performance' means the ability of a device to correctly detect or measure a particular analyte;
'clinical performance' means the ability of a device to yield results that are correlated with a particular clinical condition or a physiological or pathological process or state in accordance with the target population and intended user;

The most important parameters for analytical and clinical performance can be found in Appendix I.II.9.1., specifically 9.1.a) and b), see Tab. 16.

Tab. 16 IVDR: Parameters of Analytical and Clinical Performance acc to Ann. I.II.9.1a+b

Analytical Performance[299] **Parameters**	**Clinical Performance Parameters**[300]
analytical sensitivity	diagnostic sensitivity
analytical specificity	diagnostic specificity
trueness (bias)	positive predictive value
precision (repeatability and reproducibility)	negative predictive value
accuracy (resulting from trueness and precision)	likelihood ratio
limits of detection and quantitation	expected values in normal and affected populations

---

[298] See definitions below acc. to IVDR: Art. 2 (38), (40), (41)

[299] As a general rule analytical performance shall always be demonstrated on the basis of analytical performance studies (Annex XIII.A.1.2.2.)

[300] See definitions in IVDR: Art 2 (41); (49)-(54)

measuring range	
linearity	
cut-off, including determination of appropriate criteria for specimen collection and handling and control of known relevant endogenous and exogenous interference	
cross- reactions	

The performance data shall be obtained following a **performance evaluation plan** to include at least (Tab. 17; IVDR: Annex XIII.A.1.1.):

Tab. 17 IVDR: Minimum content of a performance evaluation plan

o *a specification of the intended purpose of the device;*
o *a specification of the characteristics of the device as described in Section 9 of Chapter II of Annex I and in point (c) of Section 20.4.1. of Chapter III of Annex I;*
o *a specification of the analyte or marker to be determined by the device;*
o *a specification of the intended use of the device;*
o *identification of certified reference materials or reference measurement procedures to allow for metrological traceability;*
o *a clear identification of specified target patient groups with clear indications, limitations and contra- indications;*
o *an identification of the general safety and performance requirements as laid down in Sections 1 to 9 of Annex I that require support from relevant scientific validity and analytical and clinical performance data;*
o *a specification of methods, including the appropriate statistical tools, used for the examination of the analytical and clinical performance of the device and of the limitations of the device and information provided by it;*
o *a description of the state of the art, including an identification of existing relevant standards, CS, guidance or best practices documents;*
o *an indication and specification of parameters to be used to determine, based on the state of the art in medicine, the acceptability of the benefit-risk ratio for the intended purpose or purposes and for the analytical and clinical performance of the device;*
o *for software qualified as a device, an identification and specification of reference databases and other sources of data used as the basis for its decision making;*
o *an outline of the different development phases including the sequence and means of determination of the scientific validity, the analytical and clinical*

> *performance, including an indication of milestones and a description of potential acceptance criteria;*
>
> o *the PMPF planning as referred to in Part B of this Annex.*

Where any of the above mentioned elements are not deemed appropriate in the Performance Evaluation Plan due to the specific device characteristics a justification shall be provided in the plan.

Performance data are mainly obtained from
(a) systematic **scientific literature review(s)** and
(b) **analytical and/or clinical performance studies** of the manufacturer;
(c) **PMPF/PMS data** out of a valid PMPF/PMS process/system

The scientific evidence from the 3 sub-reports on scientific validity, analytical and clinical performance following the path of the performance evaluation plan is summarized in the **Performance Evaluation Report (PER**; see Tab. 18[301]**)**, which is also a major part of the technical documentation according to IVDR: Annex II.6.
The performance evaluation is actively and systematically updated over the life-cycle of the IVD by **Post-Market Performance Follow-up (PMPF)**[302] based on a **PMPF plan,** exerted by **general and specific PMCF methods** and evaluated by **PMPF evaluation reports**.
For classes C + D these must be updated at least once a year.

A **Summary of Safety and Performance (SSP)** has to be drawn up by the manufacturer for classes C and D (Art. 29), the draft will be validated and then uploaded by the NB to EUDAMED.
The clinical evidence shall be documented in a **performance evaluation report**. This report shall include (Tab. 18):

Tab. 18 IVDR: Structure and Content of Performance Evaluation Report (PER)

o *the scientific validity report,*
o *the analytical performance report,*
o *the clinical performance report,*

---

[301] IVDR: Annex XIII.A.1.3.2.
[302] See details in IVDR: Annex XIII.B

o	an assessment of the reports above, allowing demonstration of the clinical evidence;
o	the justification for the approach taken to gather the clinical evidence;
o	the literature search protocol(s), incl. methodology and the report of a literature review with the full texts of the relevant articles;
o	documentation and reports of analytical and clinical performance studies;
o	the technology on which the device is based, the intended purpose of the device and any claims made about the device's performance or safety;
o	the nature and extent of the scientific validity and the analytical and clinical performance data that has been evaluated;
o	the clinical evidence as the acceptable performances against the state of the art in medicine;
o	any new conclusions derived from PMPF reports in accordance with Annex XIII.Part B[303]

---

[303] as required by IVDR: Annex XIII.A.1.3.3.

Fig. 20 IVDR: Overview Performance Evaluation Process

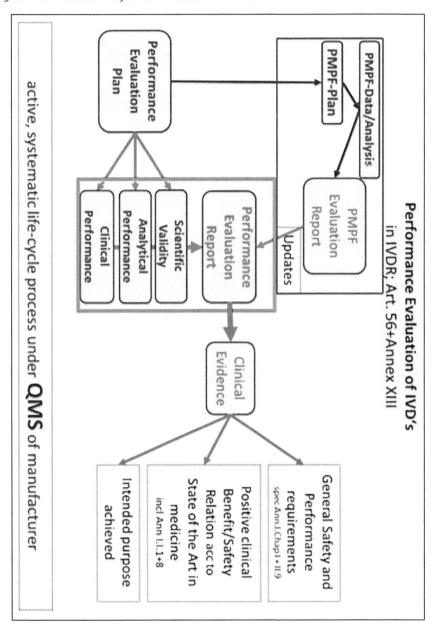

Chapter 8. Clinical investigation of medical devices

> *'clinical investigation'* *means any systematic investigation involving one or more human subjects, undertaken to assess the safety or performance of a device;*

> *'investigational device'*[304] *means a device that is assessed in a clinical investigation;*

Sources:

Legal text:

MDR: Definitions: Art. 2 No. 45-59; Main text: Chapter VI and Annex XV

Guidelines:

MDCG 2021-28: Substantial modification of clinical investigation under Medical Device Regulation

MDCG 2021-20: Instructions for generating CIV-ID for MDR Clinical Investigations

MDCG 2021-8 Clinical investigation application/notification documents

MDCG 2021-6 Regulation (EU) 2017/745 – Questions & Answers regarding clinical investigation

MDCG 2020-10/1/2: Guidance on safety reporting in clinical investigations +
Appendix: Clinical investigation summary safety report form

various MEDDEVs, to be adapted to MDR

Standards, Common Specifications (CS), other sources:

Harmonized standard: EN ISO 14155: Clinical investigation of medical devices on humans - Good clinical practice;

More and more product group specific standards now contain hints for the choice of parameters and related outcomes for clinical safety and clinical benefit for clinical investigation and clinical evaluation, e.g. within the ISO 11979-series on Intraocular lenses; ISO 81060-2 on clinical investigation of Non-invasive sphygmomanometers, the ISO 5840-series on cardiac valve prostheses or ISO/DIS 21535 on hip-joint replacement implants or ISO/DIS 21536 on knee-joint replacement implants.

It may also be useful to look into existing data banks for clinical trials, like clinicaltrials.gov[305] or WHO's International Clinical Trials Registry Platform (ICTRP)[306] or for HTA- or EbM-reports or guidances of scientific societies for inspiration.

---

[304] Also known as investigational medical device, IMD

[305] https://clinicaltrials.gov/

[306] https://www.who.int/clinical-trials-registry-platform

Clinical investigations are scientifically and ethically based clinical studies that evaluate whether a MD meets expectations or claims for clinical safety and/or clinical efficacy and/or positive clinical benefit/risk ratio under reality conditions in patients from the target groups. In view of the risks always associated with these human trials, the EU legislator sets high safety, ethical, scientific and procedural requirements for clinical investigations for the clinical evaluation in the context of conformity assessment. This has been done largely in accordance with important provisions of current EU pharmaceutical legislation[307] and provides for appropriate controls at Member State level by Ethics Committee(s) and competent authorities[308] (MDR: Chap. VI and Annex XV). For clinical investigations that do not serve the clinical evaluation in the context of conformity assessment, the MDR formulates basic safety, ethical and scientific requirements; detailed regulations, in particular with regard to eg. notifications, registration, validation, approval/non-interdiction (tacit approval) procedures, division of responsibilities between ethics committees and Competent Authorities etc. are the responsibility of the Member States.

Under the MDR, the manufacturer must control his clinical investigations from his <u>clinical evaluation plan</u> and here specifically from the <u>clinical development plan</u> (see MDR, Chapter VI and Annex XIV.A.I.a).

Besides the results of literature search and Post market clinical Follow-up (PMCF), clinical investigations are the most important source of reliable clinical data for the proof of sufficient clinical evidence for a medical device. Fig. 23 shows the main aspects to be observed, implemented and documented in clinical investigations of MDs:

1) Investigational Medical Devices, IMDs, must meet the applicable **General Safety and Performance Requirements of Annex I** of the MDR, unless these are to be established during the investigation. With regard to these aspects still to be reviewed, all necessary steps and safeguards must be taken under

---

307 REGULATION (EU) No 536/2014 OF THE EUROPEAN PARLIAMENT AND OF THE COUNCIL of 16 April 2014 on clinical trials on medicinal products for human use, and repealing Directive 2001/20/EC; see below under 3) special protection regulations
308 Division of responsibilities between Ethics Committee and Competent Authority to be decided by MS

risk management to avert any risks to subjects, users and 3rd persons[309] (see also Chapter V.1. of this book). Demonstrated technical, preclinical and previous clinical test results available for the MD will have to make it probable, that the safety and efficacy goals of the clinical investigation can be achieved in the intended study population. The essential document in this regard is the **Investigator's Brochure (IB)**. The IB should therefore demonstrate that the investigational device is safe and effective from all perspectives (from a scientific, technical, preclinical and previous clinical perspective) within the framework of the planned clinical investigation. The structure and main contents of the Investigator's Brochure can now be found in MDR: Annex XV.II.2. and in more detail in EN ISO 14155. MDCG 2021-8 "Clinical investigation application/notification documents" (including a template for a GSPR-Matrix for the IB under the MDR) is helpful guidance. Existing Device Specific Guidance (DSG) or Common Specifications (CS), once available, will have to be considered for the relevant product range.

2) Each clinical investigation shall have a sound **scientific basis**; it shall be designed in such a way that the explicitly established test hypothesis(es) can be scientifically confirmed or falsified. The key document here is the **Clinical Investigation Plan (CIP)**, which sets out the overall rationale, objectives, design, methodology, monitoring, conduct, documentation, and method of analysis for the trial. The choice of relevant parameters and related patient-relevant, measurable outcomes for clinical benefits and clinical safety and a clear definition of target groups with indications and contraindications and recruitment provisions, will also be a central task under the CIP.
The clinical evaluation plan of the manufacturer will play a key role for the CIP in the background!
The CIP is the <u>central document of the clinical investigation</u>.
The structure and main contents of the CIP can now be found in MDR: Annex XV.II.3 and in more detail in EN ISO 14155. MDCG 2021-8 "Clinical investigation application/notification documents" again is helpful guidance.
To address aspects of **(serious) adverse events and device deficiencies** during clinical investigations in the CIP, you should carefully look at MDCG 2020-

---

[309] A statement to that aspect has to be issued, see MDR: Art. 62 (4) c); Art. 71 (3) a) and Annex XV.II.4.1.

10/1/2 "Guidance on safety reporting in clinical investigations" with "Appendix: Clinical investigation summary safety report form".

Case report forms (CRF) serve the standardised clinical data collection in view of the chosen (measurable, patient-relevant) clinical parameters and related outcomes for clinical safety and/or efficacy in the subjects at the pre-defined time points of examinations and combine these with the concurrent data on the IMD and its application, if necessary.

3) **Special protection regulations** for the subjects and especially for vulnerable groups are very important in MDR: the regulations for: Informed consent (Art. 63), incapacitated subjects (Art. 64), minors (Art. 65), pregnant and breastfeeding women (Art. 66), national protective measures (Art. 67), emergency clinical investigations (Art. 68) and basic provisions for compensation (Art.69) have been largely harmonised with Regulation (EU) 2014/536 on clinical trials of pharmaceuticals and should contribute to harmonisation of the clinical research landscape in Europe. This will also facilitate combination studies.

Organisational (including role descriptions of investigator, sponsor[310] and monitor) and **general documentation issues** are described in EN ISO 14155 (and national provisions).

4) The **approval procedures** for clinical investigations, after application through EUDAMED (which also generates automatically the unique identification number[311] for this clinical investigation), include control at Member State level by the Ethics Committee(s) and competent national authorities[312]. At the sponsor's request, the procedure of separate assessment by each member state (i.e. the "classic" single Member State procedure), or the procedure of coordinated assessment (all concerned Member States assess the application in cooperation under the lead of a coordinating Member State) can be invoked.

---

[310] See the provisions for a legal representative or a contact person of the sponsor, if the sponsor is not established in the Union, in MDR: Art. 62 (2) and in national provisions of the MS

[311] See here MDCG 2021-20 "Instructions for generating CIV-ID for MDR Clinical Investigations"

[312] Division of responsibilities at the discretion of the Member State

The **classic single MS procedure** (Fig. 21) differentiates between low-risk and high-risk investigational devices, where type and intensity of control is differentiated according to the risk of IMDs [Art. 70 (7)]. The application is assessed separately by each MS.

Fig. 21 MDR Clinical Investigation single MS procedure

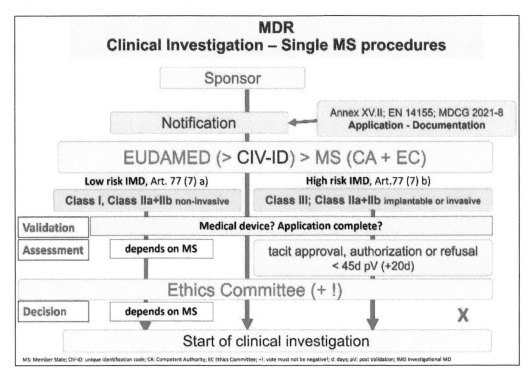

> **a) Classic single Member State procedure in the low risk area**
> (Fig. 21, left side; Class I and non-invasive IMD of Classes IIa and IIb)[313]
> Here the sponsor, at the discretion of the Member State, can start the clinical investigation after notification, code generation and successful validation, provided the Ethics Committee's opinion is not negative. This is a kind

---

[313] See MDR: Art. 70 (7) (a)

of tacit approval procedure (unless otherwise stated by national law of the Member State [314]). Phase sequence:

- **Notification** with application documents (acc. to Annex XV.II.) to EU-DAMED, generation of the unique identification number;[315]

- **Validation** within 10d[316] by Member State (examination whether the clinical investigation (the IMD) falls under the MDR and the application documents are complete).

- the **Ethics Committee** Vote must not be negative! Unless otherwise stated by national law, the sponsor may start the clinical investigation immediately after the validation.

b) Classic single Member State procedure in the high-risk area
(Fig.21, right side; Class III and invasive IMDs of Class IIa and IIb)[317]:
Approval procedure by the Member State to be completed within 45d post-validation date (+ev. further 20d). Phase sequence:

- **Notification** with application documents (acc. to Annex XV) to EU-DAMED, generation of the unique identification number;[318]

- **Validation** by Member State within 10d[319] (check whether the IMD falls under the MDR and the application documents are complete)

- **Assessment and decision** within 45 pV[320] (+ev. 20d for expert opinion); in-depth assessment of application; the vote of the **ethics committee** must not be negative! Member State may provide for appeal procedures.

---

[314] Please note that some regions, eg. in Scandinavia usually request a formal approval by the Competent Authority (CA)

[315] See here also MDCG 2021-8 "Clinical investigation application/notification documents" and MDCG 2021-20 "Instructions for generating CIV-ID for MDR Clinical Investigations"

[316] See specific timeframes in case of requests for improvements of the application in MDR: Art. 70.

[317] See MDR: Art. 70 (7) (b)

[318] See here also MDCG 2021-8 "Clinical investigation application/notification doc-uments" and MDCG 2021-20 "Instructions for generating CIV-ID for MDR Clinical Investigations"

[319] See specific timeframes in case of requests for improvements of the application

[320] pV: post Validation date

Fig. 22 MDR Clinical investigation coordinated procedure

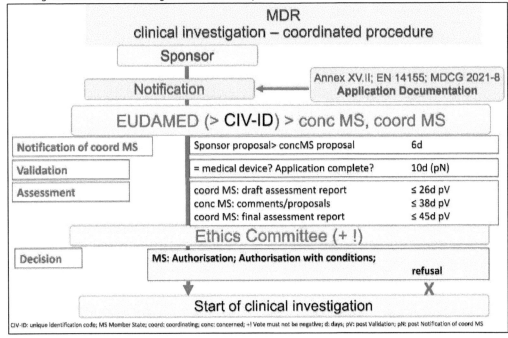

From the Date of Application (DoA) of the MDR, initially on a voluntary basis for the MSs until 27 May 2027, then compulsory at the request of the sponsor, there is the possibility of a (Fig. 22):

(c) coordinated assessment procedure[321] by all the Member States involved; this procedure shall subsequently[322] become binding on the Member States, provided that the sponsor invokes the coordinated procedure. The Member States involved work here under the leadership of a coordinating Member State, which integrates the Member States involved (concerned Member States) in the processing and evaluation of the application. The coordinating Member State is proposed by the sponsor, but ultimately determined by the Member States concerned. The following phase sequence is planned:

---

[321] See MDR: Art. 78; see also Fig. 19
[322] from 27 May 2027

Notification: application with documents acc. to Annex XV to EUDAMED, study receives the unique identification number;[323] sponsor communicates request for coordinated procedure and proposes the coordinating Member State and the Member States concerned by him; concerned Member States decide on actual coordinating Member State [324] (notification date: within 6d after application)
Validation: coordinating Member State carries out validation (= check whether IMD falls under MDR and whether documents are complete) within 10d pN[325], taking into account the comments of the MSs concerned (validation date);
Assessment: in-depth examination and evaluation of the application: the coordinating Member State prepares a draft assessment report and submits it to the Member States concerned within 26d pV; the Member States submit their comments within 38d pV, which the coordinating Member State takes into account;
The coordinating Member State prepares the final assessment report (assessment date) within 45d pV (possibly + 50d for consultation with experts for classes IIb and III), which is also considered the opinion of the Member States concerned; however, Member States may opt out (especially if their objections have not been taken into account as mentioned above; negative vote of the Ethics Committee or if e.g. national regulations would be violated). Parts of the evaluation remain reserved to the individual Member State involved[326].
Decision: Member States concerned inform the sponsor of their decision within 5d after submission of the final assessment report. (Member States provide for legal remedies)

---

[323] See here also MDCG 2021-8 "Clinical investigation application/notification doc-uments" and MDCG 2021-20 "Instructions for generating CIV-ID for MDR Clinical Investigations"

[324] If MSs concerned do not agree on a coordinating MS, the one proposed by the sponsor is taken

[325] pN: post Notification date of the coordinating Member State, as decided by the Member States concerned

[326] mainly ethical and local (clinical investigation site, clinical investigator) considerations

d) In the event of a planned **substantial modification of a clinical investigation**[327], a supplementary approval/tacit approval procedure shall be conducted following notification to EUDAMED[328]. The sponsor may enact the modification at the earliest 38d (poss. +7d) after notification, unless there is a negative vote by the ethics committee and/or there is a refusal by the Member State, based on considerations of public health, subject and user safety or health or public policy.

(e) An abridged procedure has been established for **clinical investigations of CE-marked MDs**[329] (PMCF investigation) within their approved intended purpose where there are additional invasive or burdensome procedures for subjects. This kind of clinical investigation will have to be notified to the Member State(s) concerned at least 30d prior to the start. Where there are no additional invasive or burdensome procedures in such studies on CE marked IMDs, the procedure is not defined by the MDR and is up to Member State procedures[330].

Where the clinical investigation of CE marked IMDs is assessing issues outside the scope of the intended purpose, the full procedures [see a) – c) as applicable] will have to be followed.

5) MDR has specific provisions for the **recording and reporting of (serious) adverse events and device deficiencies and the updates**[331] of these reports

---

[327] See here specifically MDCG 2021-28: "Substantial modification of clinical investigation under Medical Device Regulation"

[328] See MDR: Art. 75; an updated version of relevant documents, with changes clearly identifiable, has to be submitted to EUDAMED.

[329] See MDR: Art. 74

[330] E.g. Notification, registration, validation, ethics committee involvement, tacit approval etc.

[331] See definitions in MDR: Art. 2 (57) – (59):

'**adverse event**' means any untoward medical occurrence, unintended disease or injury or any untoward clinical signs, including an abnormal laboratory finding, in subjects, users or other persons, in the context of a clinical investigation, whether or not related to the investigational device;

'**serious adverse event**' means any adverse event that led to any of the following: (a) death, (b) serious deterioration in the health of the subject, that resulted in any of the following:
    (i) life-threatening illness or injury,
    (ii) permanent impairment of a body structure or a body function,
    (iii) hospitalization or prolongation of patient hospitalization,

as part of the clinical investigation[332]. Adverse events, identified in the CIP as critical for the benefit/risk ratio of the IMD and serious adverse events (SAE) and device deficiencies (DD) and updates to these have to be fully recorded in the documentation of the clinical investigation. SAE and DD and their updates must be reported via EUDAMED to all Member States involved. (see Fig. 23)

Please note the new MDCG Guidance: MDCG 2020-10/1/2: "Guidance on safety reporting in clinical investigations.

Appendix: Clinical investigation summary safety report form."

In the case of CE marked IMDs the vigilance reporting scheme would apply, unless a causal relationship between the SAE and the preceding clinical investigation procedures has been established, where again the specific clinical investigation reporting must be followed.

Clinical investigations started before the new MDR is applicable (26 May 2021) may be continued in accordance with Directives 93/42/EEC and 90/385/EEC. However, MDR applies to the recording and reporting of (serious) adverse events and device deficiencies and their updates, from the date of application of the new MDR (as of May 26, 2021).

6) The provisions for **termination notifications** of the clinical investigation in a Member State or in the EU/EEA, as well as the sponsor's notifications in the event of **temporary suspension or premature termination** of the clinical investigation, have now also been clearly established[333].

7) Finally, the **Clinical Investigation Report (CIR)** and a corresponding **Summary Report** must be prepared, which have to be made publicly available through EUDAMED after certain deadlines (usually 1y). The report on the clinical investigation is described in MDR: Annex XV.III.7 and specified in EN

(iv) medical or surgical intervention to prevent life-threatening illness or injury or permanent impairment to a body structure or a body function,
(v) chronic disease,
(c) fetal distress, fetal death or a congenital physical or mental impairment or birth defect;
'**device deficiency**' means any inadequacy in the identity, quality, durability, reliability, safety or performance of an investigational device, including malfunction, use errors or inadequacy in information supplied by the manufacturer;
[332] See MDR: Art. 80
[333] See MDR: Art. 77

ISO 14155. The COM can provide guidelines for the Summary Report and the possible release and presentation of raw data by the sponsor.

The new European database EUDAMED plays an important role in clinical investigation data traffic and will also generate the <u>unique clinical investigation identification number</u>[334] (clinical investigations and performance studies module). In line with the Helsinki Declaration, this should also prevent "unsuitable" clinical investigations from falling by the wayside and generating an evaluation BIAS within the framework of clinical evaluation.

---

[334] MDCG 2021-20: Instructions for generating CIV-ID for MDR Clinical Investigations

Fig. 23 MDR SAE/DD recording and reporting in clinical investigations

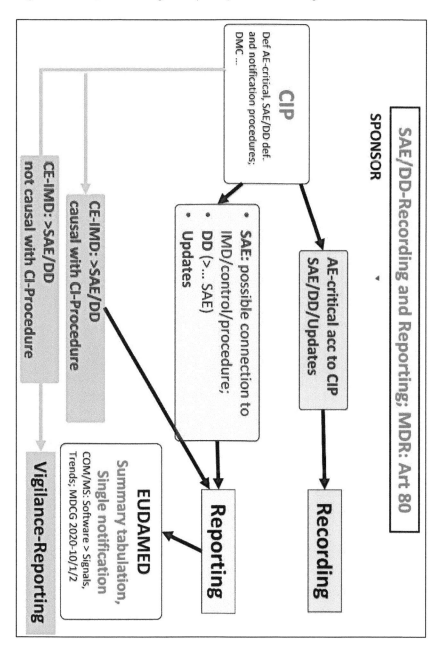

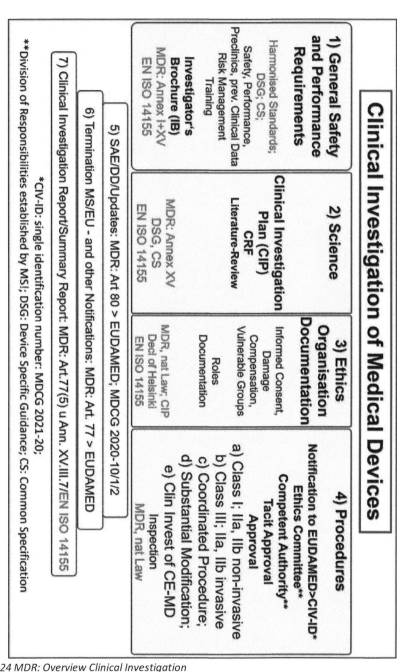

Clinical Investigation of Medical Devices

1) General Safety and Performance Requirements

Harmonised Standards;
DSG; CS;
Safety, Performance,
Preclinics, prev. Clinical Data
Risk Management
Training

Investigator's Brochure (IB)
MDR: Annex I+XV
EN ISO 14155

2) Science

Clinical Investigation Plan (CIP)
CRF
Literature-Review

MDR: Annex XV
DSG, CS
EN ISO 14155

3) Ethics Organisation Documentation

Informed Consent,
Damage Compensation,
Vulnerable Groups

Roles
Documentation

MDR, nat Law; CIP
Decl of Helsinki
EN ISO 14155

4) Procedures

Notification to EUDAMED>CIV-ID*
Ethics Committee**
Competent Authority**
Tacit Approval

a) Class I; IIa, IIb non-invasive Approval
b) Class III; IIa, IIb invasive
c) Coordinated Procedure;
d) Substantial Modification;
e) Clin Invest of CE-MD Inspection
MDR, nat Law

---

5) SAE/DD/Updates: MDR: Art 80 > EUDAMED; MDCG 2020-10/1/2

6) Termination MS/EU - and other Notifications: MDR: Art. 77 > EUDAMED

7) Clinical Investigation Report/Summary Report: MDR: Art.77(5) u Ann. XV.III.7/EN ISO 14155

*CIV-ID: single identification number: MDCG 2021-20;

**Division of Responsibilities established by MSI; DSG: Device Specific Guidance; CS: Common Specification

Fig. 24 MDR: Overview Clinical Investigation

Chapter 9. Performance studies of IVDs

> *'**performance study**' means a study undertaken to establish or confirm the analytical or clinical performance of a device;*[335]

> *'**device for performance study**' means a device intended by the manufacturer to be used in a performance study.*
> *A device intended to be used for research purposes, without any medical objective, shall not be deemed to be a device for performance study;*[336]

Sources:
IVDR: Definitions in Art. 2, (42)-(62); main text: Chapter VI and Annexes XIII.2 and XIV

Draft standard: ISO EN 20916[337]

Besides literature searches and Post market performance Follow-up (PMPF), performance studies are the most important source of clinical evidence for IVDs. These are scientific studies to clarify the analytical and/or clinical performance of IVDs. The necessity, scope and specificity of the performance studies are to be controlled by the manufacturer's **performance evaluation plan** (see chapter VII above). These studies are regulated in the IVDR largely in parallel with clinical investigations of MDs and clinical trials of pharmaceuticals[338], which will facilitate combination studies (e.g. of companion diagnostics) and harmonise the European clinical research landscape.

The basic aspects of performance studies according to the IVDR are shown in Fig. 26.

Article 57 of the IVDR defines **general requirements for all performance studies**, such as compliance with the general safety and performance requirements of Annex I, protection of the rights, safety, dignity and well-being of study subjects and ensuring the scientific soundness of study design and data collection and evaluation. In addition, data protection regulations must be observed (also) in studies with residual samples (left-over specimens).

While these requirements must be observed in all performance studies, for certain "critical" performance studies, as defined in Art. 58 (1) and (2), the

---

[335] IVDR: Art. 2 (42)
[336] IVDR: Art. 2 (45); for these research use only (RUO) products see also MEDDEV 2.14/2
[337] Still to be harmonized for IVDR
[338] See Regulation (EU) No 536/2014

procedures under section 4a)-e) in this chapter apply. For performance studies that do not fall under the procedures under 4.a)-e), it is up to the Member State to specify procedures, e.g. notification requirements, registration, validation, involvement of an ethics committee, possibly tacit approval or formal approval procedures.

Aspects 1)-3) and 5) - 7) in Fig. 26 run largely parallel to the requirements for clinical investigations of MDs (see for comparison Fig. 24):

1) Devices for performance studies must meet the applicable **general safety and performance requirements of Annex I** of the IVDR, unless these are to be established during the study. With regard to these aspects still to be reviewed, all necessary steps and safeguards must be taken under risk management to avert any risks to subjects, users and 3rd persons (see also Chapter V.1. of this book). Technical, analytical and previous clinical performance results available for the IVD will have to make it probable, that the safety and efficacy goals of the performance study can be achieved. The essential document in this regard is the **Investigator's Brochure (IB).** The IB should therefore demonstrate that the device for performance study will be safe and effective from all perspectives (from a scientific, technical, analytical and previous clinical perspective) within the framework of the planned performance study. The structure and main contents of the Investigator's Brochure can now be found in IVDR: Annex XIV.I.2 and in more detail in ISO EN 20916[339].

2) Each performance study shall have a sound **scientific basis**; it shall be designed in such a way that the explicitly established test hypothesis(es), concerning the parameters for analytical a/o clinical performance, see Tab. 16, can be scientifically confirmed or falsified. The key document here is the **Performance Study Plan (PSP)**, which sets out the overall rationale, objectives, design, methodology, monitoring, conduct, documentation, and method of analysis for the study and is therefore the central document of the performance study. The structure and main contents of the PSP can now be found in IVDR: Annex XIII.A. 2 and 3 and in more detail in ISO EN 20916.

Please note that in the case of clinical performance studies the analytical performance must have been established beforehand according to the state of

---

[339] has to be transferred into an EN and be harmonized to IVDR

the art. For interventional clinical performance studies, the analytical performance and the scientific validity must have been demonstrated according to the state of the art. Where for companion diagnostics the scientific validity is not established, the scientific rationale for the biomarker must be provided[340].

3) **Special ethical and protection provisions** for subjects and especially for vulnerable groups and subjects are highlighted in the IVDR: the provisions for: Informed consent (Art. 59), incapacitated subjects (Art. 60), minors (Art. 61), pregnant and breastfeeding women (Art. 62), national protective measures (Art. 63), emergency performance studies (Art. 64) and basic provisions for compensation (Art.65) have been largely harmonised with Regulation (EU) 2014/536 on clinical trials of pharmaceuticals and with corresponding provision of the MDR and should contribute to harmonisation of the clinical research landscape in Europe. This will also facilitate combination studies.

Organisational (including role descriptions of investigator, sponsor[341] and monitor) and **general documentation issues** will be treated in the forthcoming standard ISO EN 20916[342] (and national provisions).

4) **Specific procedures with ethics committees and competent Authorities**[343], apply for certain "critical" performance studies (see a) to e) below), in particular about tacit approval/formal approval. Procedural steps and deadlines largely correspond to the corresponding procedures in the clinical investigation of MDs.

For these studies, in addition to the general requirements of IVDR: Articles 57 and Annex XIII.A.2 and 3, the design, notification with application, validation, tacit approval/formal approval, conduct, recording and reporting of AE, SAE and DD must be carried out in accordance with IVDR: Articles 58 to 77 and Annex XIII.A.2+3 and Annex XIV.

The following procedures are described in the IVDR:

---

[340] See IVDR: Art. 58 (5) (m) and (n)
[341] See the provisions for a legal representative or a contact person, if the sponsor is not established in the Union, in IVDR: Art. 58 (4) and in national provisions of the MS
[342] This standard has to be harmonised for the IVDR
[343] Share of responsibilities between them depends on specific national provisions

a) Classical single Member State procedure with low risk[344]

(surgical invasive sampling for the purpose of the performance study, but without significant risk for subjects).

notification to EUDAMED with the application documents in Annex XIII.A.2+3 and Annex XIV (which also generates the <u>Union wide single identification number</u> for this performance study)
validation (i.e. examination whether the study falls under the IVDR and whether the application documents are complete[345])
start of the performance study possible if no negative vote of the ethics committee and unless otherwise stated by national law of Member State [346]

b) Classical single Member State procedure in the high-risk area[347]

in which a full assessment and approval procedure is carried out by each Member State concerned to be completed within 45d pV (+ev. 20d for expert consultation)

This applies to performance studies which are
- an **interventional clinical performance study**[348] or where
- the conduct of the study involves **additional invasive procedures or other risks** for the subjects, or a
- study with **companion diagnostics** (except if only residual samples are used; notification to the competent authority is required here), or
- other studies than under a)[349]

Stage sequence:
- **Notification** with application documents (acc. to Annex XIII.A. 2+3; Annex XIV) to EUDAMED, generation of the unique identification number;
- **Validation** by Member State within 10d[350] (check whether study falls under the IVDR and the application documents are complete)
- **Assessment and decision**[351] within 45 pV[352] (+poss. 20d for expert opinion); in-depth assessment of application; the vote of the **ethics committee** must not be negative! Member State may provide for appeal procedures.

---

[344] See IVDR: Art. 66 (7) a)

[345] acc. to Annex XIII.A.2+3 and Annex XIV

[346] Some MS might require a formal approval of studies in any case

[347] See IVDR: Art. 66 (7) b)

[348] Definition see IVDR, Art. 2 no. 46

[349] This reference seems unclear and might necessitate official interpretation

[350] See specific timeframes in case of requests for improvements of the application

[351] Work share between Competent Authority and Ethics Committee determined by MS!

[352] pV: post Validation date

In addition, from the date of application of the IVDR (25 May 2022) until 27 May 2029 on a voluntary basis for Member States and later compulsory at the request of the sponsor, there will be the possibility of a

(c) coordinated procedure[353] by all the Member States involved; this procedure can be invoked by the sponsor. The Member States involved work here under the leadership of a <u>coordinating Member State</u>, which integrates the Member States involved (<u>concerned Member States</u>) in the processing and evaluation of the application. The coordinating Member State is proposed by the sponsor, but ultimately determined by the Member States concerned. The following phase sequence is planned:

Notification: application with documents acc. to Annex XIII.A.2+3 and Annex XIV to EUDAMED, study receives the unique identification number; sponsor communicates request for coordinated procedure and proposes the coordinating Member State and the Member States concerned; concerned Member States decide on actual coordinating Member State[354] (<u>notification date</u>: within 6d after application)

Validation: coordinating Member State carries out validation (= check whether study falls under IVDR and whether documents are complete) within 10d pN[355], taking into account the comments of the Member States concerned (<u>validation date</u>);

Assessment: in-depth examination and evaluation of the application: the coordinating Member State prepares a <u>draft assessment report</u> and submits it to the Member States concerned within 26d pV; the Member States submit their comments within 38d pV, which the coordinating Member State takes into account; the coordinating Member State prepares the <u>final assessment report</u> (<u>assessment date</u>) within 45d pV (possibly + 50d for consultation with experts for classes C and D), which is also considered the opinion of the Member States concerned; however, Member States may opt out (especially if their objections have not been taken into account as mentioned above; negative vote of the Ethics Committee or if e.g. national regulations would be violated). Parts of the evaluation remain reserved to the individual Member State involved[356].

---

[353] See IVDR: Art. 74

[354] In case the Member States concerned do not agree, the Member State proposed by the sponsor will be the coordinating Member State

[355] pN: post Notification date of the coordinating MS, as decided by the MSs concerned; in case of requests for improvement of application see timeframes in Art. 74 (4) c) [ref. to Art. 66 (3)-(5)]

[356] mainly ethical and local: (performance study site, investigator) considerations

> **Decision**: Member States concerned inform the sponsor of their decision within 5d after submission of the final assessment report. (Member States provide for legal remedies)

d) In the event of a planned **substantial modification of a performance study**, a supplementary approval/tacit approval procedure shall be conducted following notification to EUDAMED[357]. The sponsor may enact the modification at the earliest 38d (ev. +7d) after notification, unless there is a negative vote by the ethics committee and/or there is a refusal by the Member State, based on considerations of public health, subject and user safety or health or public policy.

(e) An abridged procedure has been established for **performance studies of CE-marked IVDs[358] (PMPF study)** within their approved intended purpose where there are additional invasive or burdensome procedures for subjects. This kind of performance study will have to be notified to the Member State (s) concerned at least 30d prior to the start. Where there are no additional invasive or burdensome procedures in such studies on CE marked IVDs, the procedure is not defined by the MDR and is up to Member State procedures[359].

Where the performance study of CE marked IVDs is assessing issues outside the scope of the intended purpose, the full procedures [see 4.a) – c) as applicable] will have to be followed.

To 5): The obligation to **record and report (serious) adverse events and device deficiencies and their updates[360]** largely corresponds to the clinical investigations of MDs (for IVDR see Fig. 25). Adverse events (AE), identified in the Performance Study Plan (PSP) as critical for the benefit/risk ratio of the product for performance study and serious adverse events (SAE) and device deficiencies (DD) and updates to these have to be fully recorded in the documentation of the performance study. SAE and DD and their updates must

---

[357] See MDR: Art. 75; an updated version of relevant documents, with changes clearly identifiable, has to be submitted to EUDAMED.

[358] See IVDR: Art. 70

[359] Eg. Notification, registration, validation, ethics committee involvement, tacit approval etc.

[360] See definitions of AE, SAE and DD in IVDR: Art. 2 (60) – (62)

be reported via EUDAMED to all Member States involved. Also the procedure for reporting these events in performance studies of CE marked IVDs is similar to MDR.

6) The provisions for **termination notifications** of the performance study in a Member State or in the EU/EEA, as well as the sponsor's notifications in the event of **temporary suspension or premature termination** of the performance study, have now also been clearly established[361].

7) Finally, the **Performance Study Report (PSR)** and a corresponding **Summary Report** must be prepared, which have to be made publicly available through EUDAMED after certain deadlines (usually 1y). The report on the performance study is described in IVDR: Annex XIII.A.2.3.3. and A.3. and specified in ISO EN 20916. The COM can provide guidelines for the Summary Report and the possible release and presentation of raw data by the sponsor.

The new European database EUDAMED plays an important role in the administrative management of performance studies and also generates the unique identification number of the performance study (module Clinical Investigations and Performance Studies). In line with the Helsinki Declaration, this registration in advance should also prevent "inappropriate" performance studies from falling by the wayside and generating a performance evaluation BIAS.

---

[361] See IVDR: Art. 73

Fig. 25 SAE/DD Recording and reporting under IVDR Performance studies

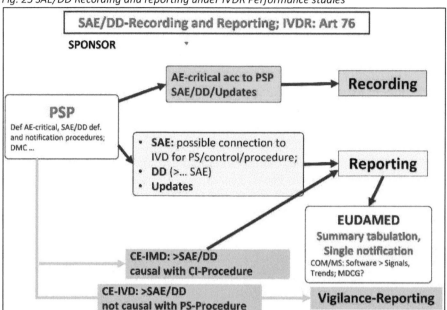

Fig. 26 IVDR: Overview Performance Studies of IVDs

Performance Studies of IVDs under IVDR
Chapt. VI + Annexes XIII.A.2 and XIV

1) General Safety and Performance Requirements

Harmonised Standards
DSG; CS;
Safety, Scientific Validity
Analyt/Clinical
Performance
Risk Management
Training

Investigator's Brochure (IB)
IVDR: Annex I+XIV
ISO EN 20916

2) Science

(Clinical) Performance Study Plan (C)PSP
Literature-Review

IVDR: Annex XIII.A.2./XIV
DSG, CS
ISO EN 20916

3) Ethics Organisation Documentation

Informed Consent,
Damage Compensation,
Vulnerable Groups

• Roles
• Documentation

IVDR, nat Law; CPSP
Decl of Helsinki
ISO EN 20916

4) Procedures
Notification to EUDAMED > ID*
Ethics Committee**
Competent Authority

a) 1-MS: surgic invas sample taking w/o risk
b) 1-MS: high risk:
• intervent.clin. PS
• additi invas Proc or other Risks for subj.
• Companion diagnostics
• Other PS than a)
c) Coordinated Procedure
d) Substantial Modification;
e) PS of CE-IVD

Tacit Approval
IVDR, nat Law

5) SAE/DD/Updates: Notifications: IVDR: Art 76 > EUDAMED

6) Termination- and other Notifications: IVDR: Art. 77 > EUDAMED

7) Performance Study Report/Summary report: IVD-V: Art.73(5) + Ann. XIV/ISO/DIS 20916

PS: Performance Study; *ID: Single identification number for PS; **Responsibilities given by MS; DSG: Device Specific
Guidance; CS: Common Specification; subj.: subjects; MS: Member State of EU/EEA; most important documents

203

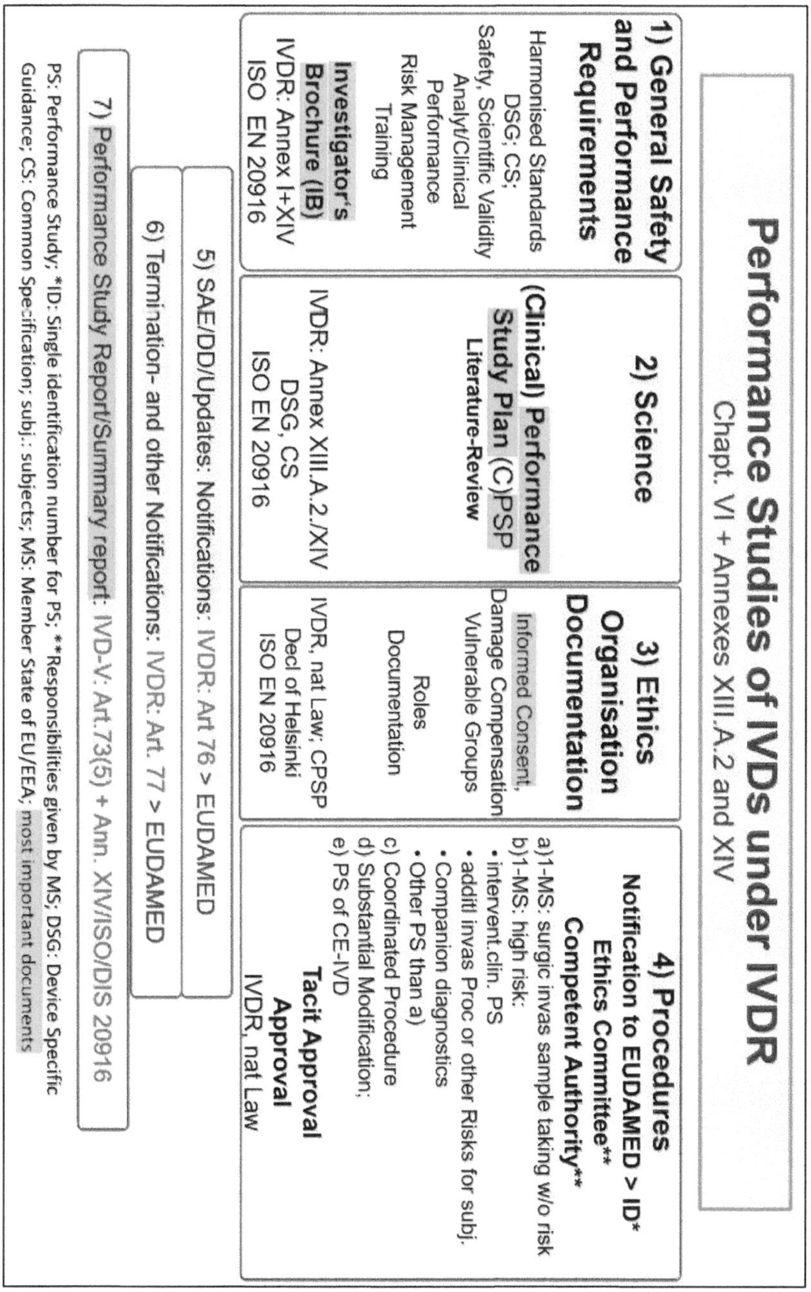

Chapter 10. Technical Documentation (TD)

Source:

Annexes II and III (PMS) of both Regulations

An important aid for manufacturers and NBs has now been provided in both regulations with the detailed presentation of the minimum contents of the technical documentation in the annexes II.

As part of the general manufacturer's obligations pursuant to Art. 10, the manufacturer must prepare and keep up to date the technical documentation in accordance with Annex II and III (PMS) of the respective Regulation for the MDs/IVDs manufactured by him[362].

This is the manufacturer's most important documentation in the MD/IVD area:

This technical documentation must allow an assessment of the conformity of the MD/IVD and of important related processes with the requirements of the respective Regulation and must be structured and detailed accordingly.

The minimum contents of the technical documentation (TD) are specified in Annex II of the respective Regulation; the technical documentation for post-market surveillance (PMS) is dealt with in Annex III (see chapter XV on PMS in this book). Fig. 27 gives an overview of the structure of both Annexes II.

(Again, a GHTF/IMDRF guideline on Summary TEchnical Documentation (STED) has largely been the inspiration here for the Annexes II).

IMDRF also offers a much more detailed version of a technical documentation for international regulatory submission purposes for MDs[363] and IVDs[364], which MDR and IVDR did not follow)

---

[362] Except for custom made devices of MDR, where a documentation acc. to Annex XIII.2 has to be provided

[363] Non-In Vitro Diagnostic Device Market Authorization Table of Contents (nIVDMAToC) http://www.imdrf.org/docs/imdrf/final/technical/imdrf-tech-190321-nivd-dma-toc-n9.pdf

[364] In Vitro Diagnostic Medical Device Market Authorization Table of Contents (IVD MA ToC) http://www.imdrf.org/docs/imdrf/final/technical/imdrf-tech-190321-ivd-mdma-toc-n13.pdf

Fig. 27 MDR/IVDR: Overview of Technical Documentation Structure

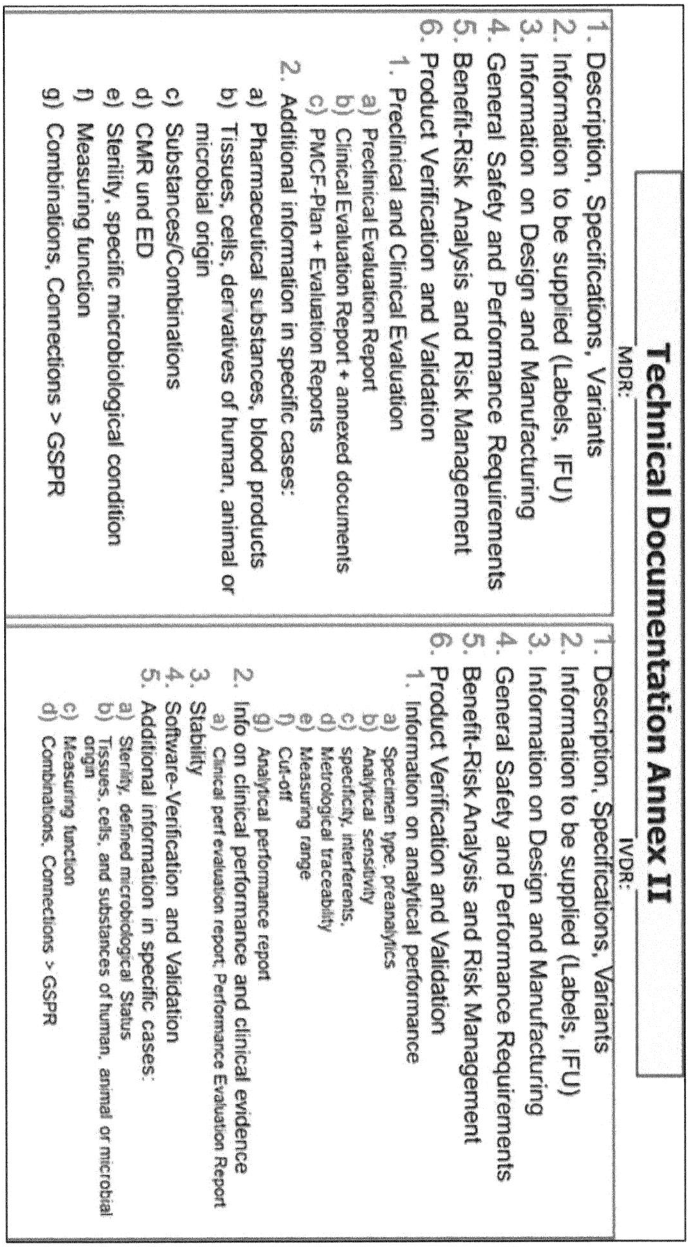

Technical Documentation Annex II

MDR:

1. Description, Specifications, Variants
2. Information to be supplied (Labels, IFU)
3. Information on Design and Manufacturing
4. General Safety and Performance Requirements
5. Benefit-Risk Analysis and Risk Management
6. Product Verification and Validation
   1. Preclinical and Clinical Evaluation
      a) Preclinical Evaluation Report
      b) Clinical Evaluation Report + annexed documents
      c) PMCF-Plan + Evaluation Reports
   2. Additional information in specific cases:
      a) Pharmaceutical substances, blood products
      b) Tissues, cells, derivatives of human, animal or microbial origin
      c) Substances/Combinations
      d) CMR und ED
      e) Sterility, specific microbiological condition
      f) Measuring function
      g) Combinations, Connections > GSPR

IVDR:

1. Description, Specifications, Variants
2. Information to be supplied (Labels, IFU)
3. Information on Design and Manufacturing
4. General Safety and Performance Requirements
5. Benefit-Risk Analysis and Risk Management
6. Product Verification and Validation
   1. Information on analytical performance
      a) Specimen type, preanalytics
      b) Analytical sensitivity
      c) specificity, interferents,
      d) Metrological traceability
      e) Measuring range
      f) Cut-off
      g) Analytical performance report
   2. Info on clinical performance and clinical evidence
      a) Clinical perf evaluation report, Performance Evaluation Report
   3. Stability
   4. Software-Verification and Validation
   5. Additional information in specific cases:
      a) Sterility, defined microbiological Status
      b) Tissues, cells, and substances of human, animal or microbial origin
      c) Measuring function
      d) Combinations, Connections > GSPR

10.1. Technical documentation for MDs

MDR: Annex II and III (PMS)

The technical Documentation (TD) has to be presented in a clear, organised, readily searchable and unambiguous manner and shall include in particular the structure and elements listed in Annex II:

1. DEVICE DESCRIPTION AND SPECIFICATION, INCLUDING VARIANTS AND ACCESSORIES

1. Device description and specification

(a) product or trade name and a general description of the device including its intended purpose[365] and intended users;

(b) the Basic UDI-DI as referred to in Part C of Annex VI assigned by the manufacturer to the device in question, as soon as identification of this device becomes based on a UDI system, or otherwise a clear identification by means of product code, catalogue number or other unambiguous reference allowing traceability; (see also Art. 27 (7): As part of the technical documentation referred to in Annex II, the manufacturer shall keep up-to-date a list of all UDIs that it has assigned.)

(c) the intended patient population and medical conditions to be diagnosed, treated and/or monitored and other considerations such as patient selection criteria, indications, contraindications, warnings;

(d) principles of operation of the device and its mode of action, scientifically demonstrated if necessary;

(e) the rationale for the qualification of the product as a device;

(f) the risk class of the device and the justification for the classification rule(s) applied in accordance with Annex VIII;

(g) an explanation of any novel features;

(h) a description of the accessories for a device, other devices and other products that are not devices, which are intended to be used in combination with it;

(i) a description or complete list of the various configurations/variants of the device that are intended to be made available on the market;

(j) a general description of the key functional elements, e.g. its parts/components (including software if appropriate), its formulation, its composition, its functionality and, where relevant, its qualitative and quantitative composition.

---

[365] Details see below

Where appropriate, this shall include labelled pictorial representations (e.g. diagrams, photographs, and drawings), clearly indicating key parts/components, including sufficient explanation to understand the drawings and diagrams;

(k) a description of the raw materials incorporated into key functional elements and those making either direct contact with the human body or indirect contact with the body[366], e.g., during extracorporeal circulation of body fluids;

(l) technical specifications, such as features, dimensions and performance attributes, of the device and any variants/configurations and accessories that would typically appear in the product specification made available to the user, for example in brochures, catalogues and similar publications.

From the product description, including its intended purpose and its (main) mechanism of action, it must be possible, to determine at least the following:

- to clarify the qualification of the product as an MD (incl. deemed to be MD: accessory, Annex XVI-product etc.);

- which general safety and performance requirements apply to the MD or not (e.g. chemical/physical/technical specifications, release of CMR substances or endocrine disruptors; possible release of nanoparticles; microbial status or reprocessibility; drug components; non-viable components of human, animal or microbial origin; possible combinations with other MDs and interactions with the environment; reusable; diagnostic or measuring functions, allowing direct diagnosis; release of ionising/non-ionising radiation; presence of programmable electronic systems (MDSW or software, which drives a device or influences the use of a device); presence of an active or active implantable MD; particular mechanical or thermal risks; risks due to release of energy or substances; lay use);

- which classification rules apply (e.g. intended type and duration of use; (not) active?; software components and their functionality(ies); regarding release of nanoparticles; diagnostic significance (direct diagnosis?); is rule 21 of Annex VIII with regard to substances applicable?

- whether consultation procedures are to be carried out for the purposes of conformity assessment (see Chapter XII.7. in this book);

---

[366] See here also the chapter on preclinical evaluation in chapter 5.4. of this book

For the description of the intended purpose, it is also important to keep in mind its definition[367]:

> *'intended purpose'* means the use for which a device is intended according to the data supplied by the manufacturer on the label, in the instructions for use or in promotional or sales materials or statements and as specified by the manufacturer in the clinical evaluation;

What is important here is above all that the determination of the intended purpose:

- is the responsibility and privilege of the manufacturer;
- is made unambiguously, consistently and without contradiction in the manufacturer's documentation and information materials; and
- is determined by the clinical evaluation and its results in terms of content and scope (especially in the case of medical purpose limitation)!

It is also useful to have the following 4 W-questions in mind, when detailing the intended purpose of the MD:

WHO should use the medical device on/for WHOM, for WHICH modalities of use, and WHY?

Tab. 19 4W Questions to specify intended purpose for MDs

1) WHO should use the MD?
- Intended users (use by health professionals/ lay persons/ persons with handicaps/disabilities; specific qualifications or specific characteristics of users required, given by specific inclusion/exclusion criteria, if applicable; Specific education or training? (simulator training?)

2) On/for WHOM is the MD to be used?
- This refers to the intended target (patient) populations (demographic characteristics such as age, gender, ethnicity, etc..., e.g. adults/children/infants, newborns, pregnant or lactating women; women of childbearing age; very old people; other vulnerable populations; general or specific health-related criteria, populations with specified general health status; with or without (certain) comorbidities or specific medical treatment history [e.g. treatment resistance?]; aspects of frailty; other aspects); specific indications or contraindications, see below.
- precise medical indications (if applicable)
- Any contraindications; further restrictions and warnings, if any.

---

[367] Art. 2 (12)

3) WHICH modalities of use of the MD are intended by the manufacturer?

The following details are of particular importance:

- Type of contact with the human body (which organs, tissues, cells, body fluids or gases; direct or indirect or no contact); contact via intact skin or mucosa; injured skin or mucosa; natural or artificial orifices; routes of inhalation; invasive, surgically invasive procedures; implantable MD;
- Duration of use or contact with the body (temporary, short-term, long-term; implantable; single, repeated or continuous use) ;
- Single use/reuse; repeat uses, including restrictions on the number or duration of repeat uses;
- Whether the MD is to be used in conjunction with specific accessories, other MDs (active, non-active), in combination with other products or treatments; whether the MD is to be used in contact with medicinal products or tissues, cells, derivatives of biological origin intended to be delivered to or removed from the human body.
- Whether the information provided by the MD to the physician will be important or crucial for (direct) diagnosis (including predictive or prognostic) or supportive; importance for patient management or public health or (individual) therapeutic purposes ;
- precautions required by the manufacturer;
- other aspects, e.g. related to procedural aspects of the use of the MD (e.g. catheter-based or minimally invasive procedures; in the context of dialysis, plasmapheresis, anaesthesia, etc).
- Application environment
- Application scenarios
- specific hardware/operating system/software environments for MDSW

4) WHY is the MD to be used on these individuals?

This question clearly refers to the stated medical purpose(s) of the MD. The possible range would correspond to the broad groups of specific medical purposes stated in the definition of a "medical device" (and not related to IVDs):

- Diagnosis, prevention, monitoring, prediction, prognosis, treatment or alleviation of disease,
- Diagnosis, monitoring, treatment, alleviation or compensation of injury or disability,
- examination, replacement or modification of the anatomy or of a physiological or pathological process or condition.

These rather broad and vague elements in the definition now need to be highly specified to really differentiate the intended medical use.

The following details for the specific medical purposes are at least expected here:

- Name of disease or condition/clinical form (e.g. acute, sub-acute, chronic, intermittent), stage (e.g. NYHA[368] I-IV), phase, severity, symptoms (e.g. pain, itching, angina

---

[368] New York Heart Association stage I-IV of heart insufficiency

209

pectoris; tremor, sweating) or other aspects to be treated, rehabilitated or diagnosed, etc.; in any case, the highly specified medical areas of use, organs, parts of the body, pathologies, (patho-)physiologies, diseases, symptoms, severities, etc. should be stated in relation to the specific medical device;

- the statements regarding the nature, extent, duration and likelihood of the claimed clinical benefit/performance and the clinical safety parameters, risks including adverse reactions, which translate into the appropriate parameters and outcomes studied for the clinical benefit/performance and clinical safety/risks (see below).

In addition, the intended use of "deemed to be medical devices" such as accessories, MDs for contraception; MDs for cleaning/disinfection/sterilisation of MDs, etc., as well as the non-medical purposes of Annex XVI devices should be considered;

The WHY also includes the precise characterisation of the principal mode or modalities of action, with a detailed description of the interaction of the MD with the human body.

- interaction of the MD with the human body (reciprocal effects on human body parts, specific organs, tissues or (patho)physiological conditions/processes; direct, indirect or no contact with patient or user) and/or the

- MD interaction with patient data (e.g. in imaging procedures for diagnostic, predictive or prognostic purposes) , telemedicine etc;

- MD interaction with patient management [e.g. surgery; anaesthesia; dialysis; plasmapheresis; proper administration of medicines, including medical gases]; telemedicine etc; and/or the

- MP interaction with public health purposes [e.g. in screening programmes or in mother-child care or protection against transmission of pathogens];

The mode(s) of action should be supported by a scientifically sound rationale, how the services/functionalities/performances of the MD can achieve the specified medical purpose(s) and an acceptable clinical benefit/risk profile in the target patient population(s) and how this could be verified with reference to the clinical evaluation of the MD (see Annex II. 6 or point 6 below).

2) Information to be supplied by the manufacturer

A complete set of:

— the label or labels on the device and on its packaging, such as single unit packaging, sales packaging, transport packaging in case of specific management conditions, in the languages accepted in the Member States where the device is envisaged to be sold; and

— the instructions for use in the languages accepted in the Member States where the device is envisaged to be sold.

Labelling and instructions for use are described very precisely in MDR: Appendix I.III.23 and the sub-items there must be processed exactly, if applicable.

Please consider also: Commission Implementing Regulation (EU) 2021/2226 of 14 December 2021 laying down rules for the application of Regulation (EU) 2017/745 of the European Parliament and of the Council as regards **electronic instructions for use** of medical devices[369]

See also EN ISO 20417 (Medical devices — Information to be supplied by the manufacturer) and EN ISO 15223-1: (Medical devices — Symbols to be used with medical device labels, labelling and information to be supplied — Part 1: General requirements).

Product and product-group specific standards may also contain additional and specific elements for label and instructions for use.

Additional information is to be delivered for Class III products and implants via the Summary of Safety and Clinical Performance (SSCP)[370]. For many Implants, Information acc. to Art. 18[371] will be necessary.

3) Information on design and manufacture[372]:

(a) information to allow the design stages applied to the device to be understood;

(b) complete information and specifications, including the manufacturing processes and their validation, their adjuvants, the continuous monitoring and the final product testing. Data shall be fully included in the technical documentation;

(c) identification of all sites, including suppliers and sub-contractors, where design and manufacturing activities are performed; Information about all design phases;

---

[369] https://eur-lex.europa.eu/eli/reg_impl/2021/2226/oj
[370] MDCG 2019-9: Summary of safety and clinical performance
[371] MDCG 2021-11: Guidance on Implant Card – Device types and MDCG 2019-8 rev2: Guidance document implant card on the application of Article 18 Regulation (EU) 2017/745 on medical devices
[372] Documentation acc. to the QMS and to EN ISO 13485 will be essential in that respect

4) General Safety and Performance Requirements (GSPR) referred to in Annex I

(see also chapter V in this book and Figs. 16 to 18)

Annex I, Chap. I ("**General requirements**") will best be worked through with (a precise reference) to the documentation of the **clinical evaluation** (see X.1.6.) below and chapter VI in this book) and (a precise reference to) the documentation of the **risk management** system (see point 5 below and chapter V.1. and Fig. 14 in this book).

For Chapter II of Annex I ("**Requirements Regarding Design and Manufacture**"), it is recommended that these sections and sub-items are systematically walked through using the 4-step procedure in Fig. 16 or a similar procedure[373]:

1. Does the GSPR (incl. sub-items) apply/not apply to the MD (with explanation)?
2. If a GSPR (incl. sub-items) applies, can compliance with it be demonstrated by presumptions of conformity in Harmonised Standard(s) and/or CS or by reference to alternative solutions (often state of the art standards, mainly from ISO or IEC) with reasoned explanation(s)?
3. Validation and verification with evidence through controlled documents (e.g. test reports, certificates, etc) as part of the TD;
4. Concluding assessment for each section of GSPR and sub-item, whether compliance is given by non-applicability or documented evidence under 3 above;

Chapter III of Annex I ("**Requirements Regarding Information supplied with the device**") is dealt with by meticulously working through section 23 (MDR) and the sub-items of this section that apply to the MD (see also point 2 above).

5) Benefit-Risk analysis and risk management

(see Chapter V.1. and Fig. 14 in this book) In addition to the description of the Risk Management System in Chapter I of Annex I, the verification must also include the risk management relating to the sections and sub-items of

---

[373] See here specifically an Annex of MDCG 2021-8: Clinical investigation application/notification documents, which provides a GSPR-Matrix in Word-format!

Chapters II and III of Annex I. This should be done with a more detailed presentation of how the minimisation principle "as far as possible" in Annex I.I.2[374] has been exerted specifically through the sections and sub-items of Chapter II of Annex I. For chapter III of Annex I a careful step-by-step walk through will be necessary.

Broad reliance should be on EN ISO 14971 and ISO TR 24971 and on some more specific standards pursuing explicitly a risk management concept[375].

6) Verification and Validation of the MD
Preclinical and clinical data (preclinical and clinical evaluation, incl. PMCF).
a) **Preclinical evaluation**: includes (MDR: Annex II.6.1.[376])
(a) results of tests, such as engineering, laboratory, simulated use and animal tests, and evaluation of published literature applicable to the device, taking into account its intended purpose, or to similar devices, regarding the pre-clinical safety of the device and its conformity with the specifications;
(b) detailed information regarding test design, complete test or study protocols, methods of data analysis, in addition to data summaries and test conclusions re-garding in particular:
— the biocompatibility of the device including the identification of all materials in direct or indirect contact with the patient or user;
— physical, chemical and microbiological characterisation;
— electrical safety and electromagnetic compatibility;
— software verification and validation (describing the software design and develop-ment process and evidence of the validation of the software, as used in the finished device. This information shall typically include the summary results of all verifica-tion, validation and testing performed both in-house and in a simulated or actual user environment prior to final release. It shall also address all of the different hard-ware configurations and, where applicable, operating systems identified in the in-formation supplied by the manufacturer);
— stability, including shelf life; and
— performance and safety.

---

[374] MDR: Annex I.I.2: The requirement in this Annex I to reduce risks as far as possible means the reduction of risks as far as possible without adversely affecting the benefit-risk ratio.
[375] Like EN ISO 10993-series; EN ISO 18562-series; EN ISO 24442-series; etc.
[376] See also chapter 5.4. in this book

Where applicable, conformity with the provisions of Directive 2004/10/EC of the European Parliament and of the Council (GLP – Good Laboratory Practice) shall be demonstrated.

Where no new testing has been undertaken, the documentation shall incorporate a rationale for that decision. An example of such a rationale would be that biocompatibility testing on identical materials was conducted when those materials were incorporated in a previous version of the device that has been legally placed on the market or put into service;

See here chapter V.4. in this book on preclinical evaluation with the documentation and the reasoning mentioned there.

Preclinical evaluation includes the literature search of the scientific pre-clinical literature and the evaluation, analysis, and if necessary, generation of pre-clinical data and documentation to prove conformity with the relevant requirements in Annex I.II, in particular Section 10 (Chemical, physical and biological properties, biocompatibility - biological evaluation), with discussion of poss. alternatives; Section 12 (pharmaceuticals and substances/combinations of substances) and Section 13 (MD with materials of biological origin) must also be examined here in coordination with the risk management.

ISO/DIS 10993-1 Annex A, Table A.1 "Endpoints to be addressed in a biological risk assessment" is a good starting point for planning and analysing the relevant requirement profile of biological evaluation for an MD[377]. It contains a matrix of the endpoints of biological evaluation to be discussed, depending on the type, intensity and duration of body contact, which, if necessary, must be processed and documented in accordance with certain standards of the EN ISO 10993 series by literature search and/or own investigations and/or presumptions of conformity from Harmonised Standards or CS or references to available data of an equivalent MD or references to an alternative solution which has to be fully justified.

---

[377] Please look also for EN ISO 18562-series for biocompatibility in the airways and ISO 7405 for biocompatibility in dentistry

The basis is always the chemical/ physical characterization of the MD[378] and the verification of the corresponding specifications.

Own investigations, tests, simulations etc. are to be presented with detailed information on test setup, complete test or study protocols, methods of data analysis, in addition to data summaries and test results; if applicable, compliance with **GLP Directive 2004/10/EC (Good Laboratory Practice)** must be demonstrated.

The NB must take into account the results of literature searches and all validations, verifications and tests carried out, as well as the conclusions drawn from them.

The manufacturer's considerations regarding the **use of alternative materials and substances, possibly other designs** (e.g. different surface textures), as well as the packaging and stability, including the shelf life of the finished product, must also be documented and justified. If a manufacturer has not carried out any new tests or if deviations from the procedures have resulted, a justification shall be provided.

With regard to Section 10 of Annex I and its documentation, the **problem of CMR-ED** (see Chapter V.3 in this book and Annex I.II.10.4 of the MDR) must be particularly taken into account, as well as the reference to the opinions of the Scientific Committee (e.g. on phthalates[379] and, if applicable, other groups of substances).

b) For **clinical evaluation**, the clinical evaluation report (CER; with annexed documents, see Tab. 13 and chapter VI in this book), the clinical evaluation plan and the PMCF plan, including PMCF evaluation reports are part of the TD.

The clinical evaluation is practically the "final validation" of the medical device with regard to the acceptability of the benefit/risk ratio against the

---

[378] See here EN ISO 10993-18, 19 and 22 (nanomaterials) for reference.

[379] Please look for SCHEER Guideline: Guidelines on the benefit-risk assessment of the presence of phthalates in certain medical devices https://ec.europa.eu/health/md_sector/new_regulations/guidance_en
covering phthalates which are carcinogenic, mutagenic, toxic to reproduction (CMR) or have endocrine-disrupting (ED) properties

medical state of the art[380]. Thus, this aspect is one of the most important parts of the technical documentation!

Save time and avoid any audit delays due to additional requests by NBs or Competent Authorities for clinical data. (It is now very easy to do this electronically!) Especially with regard to your clinical investigations, relevant documents such as CIP (Clinical Investigation Plan), IB (Investigator's Brochure), CIR (Clinical Investigation Report) and Summary Report, statements from the ethics committee(s) and competent authority(ies) involved should be annexed. With regard to the literature searches, Literature search protocol(s) and Literature search report(s), as well as the full texts of the relevant literature[381] should be annexed. According to the MDR, the NBs must assess the clinical dossiers in the context of the conformity assessment now much more intensely and professionally. They have significantly expanded and qualified their personnel capacities for this purpose! NBs will have to issue the obligatory Clinical Evaluation Assessment Report [CEAR][382] on their clinical assessment activities of the MD concerned.

Additional documentation required in specific cases:
a) MDs with pharmaceutical components:
[MD incorporates, as an integral part a substance, which, if used separately, may be considered to be a medicinal product within the meaning of point 2 of Article 1 of Directive 2001/83/EC, including a medicinal product derived from human blood or human plasma, as referred to in the first subparagraph of MDR: Art. 1(8)]. In these cases, the documentation shall include an exact indication of the source of the substance (even if derived from human blood or plasma) and the data from the tests carried out considering the intended use of the product to assess its safety, quality and usefulness by analogy with the methods described in Annex I of Directive 2001/83/EC.
See also: MEDDEV 2.1/3, currently under revision;

---

[380] personal communication by Gerold Labek, Chairman of EARN (European Arthroplasty Register Network)
[381] insofar as not already included directly in the CER
[382] See MDCG 2020-13: Clinical evaluation assessment report template

EMA Assessment templates and guidance - Ancillary medicinal substances incorporated in a medical device: https://www.ema.europa.eu/en/human-regulatory/overview/medical-devices

These sources will also help you getting the documentation right for a consultation procedure according to MDR: Annex IX.II.5.2 or Annex X.6, where the quality, safety and usefulness of the substance must be verified by analogy with the methods specified in Annex I to Directive 2001/83/EC.[383]

(b) (non-viable) components of human or animal origin:

Non-viable components of human origin: these components must be declared.

MD with non-viable component of human origin in ancillary function acc. to Art. 1 (10), 1st subpara: for MDs containing such components the provisions for donation, procurement and testing laid down in Directive 2004/23/EC apply and relevant documentation must be provided.

MDs according to Art. 1 (6) g)[384]: In this case, the documentation contains the exact details of all materials used of human origin and detailed information on conformity with section 13.1. of Annex I (see also chapter 5.3. in this book, including the reference to the error in section 13 of Annex I.II. of MDR).

Non-viable components of animal origin: these components must be declared.

MDs according to Art. 1 (6) f): In this case, the documentation contains the exact details of all materials used of animal[385] origin and detailed information on conformity with section 13.2. of Annex I (see also chapter 5.3. in this book)

---

[383] See general EMA Guidances for the interface between MDs, IVDs and pharmaceuticals: https://www.ema.europa.eu/en/human-regulatory/overview/medical-devices

[384] *however this Regulation does apply to devices manufactured utilising derivatives of tissues or cells of human origin which are non-viable or are rendered non-viable;*

[385] For the prevention of Transmissible Spongiform Encephalopathies (TSE): See Commission Regulation (EU) No 722/2012 of 8 August 2012 concerning particular requirements as regards the requirements laid down in Council Directives 90/385/EEC and 93/42/EEC with respect to active implantable medical devices and medical devices manufactured utilising tissues of animal origin. Please note that this Regulation under Directives 93/42/EEC and 90/385/EEC is now also an implementing Regulation under the MDR. A Specific Evaluation Report of the NB (SER) has to be sent to the Competent Authorities of the EU for scrutiny (see chapter 13.9 for consultation procedure)

(c) Substances/combinations of substances:

For products consisting of substances or combinations of substances intended to be introduced into the human body and absorbed by the human body or distributed locally in the body, detailed information, including test set-up, complete test or study protocols, methods of data analysis and data summaries and test results related to studies on:

- absorption, distribution, metabolism and excretion;
- possible interactions of these substances or their metabolites in the human body with other products, medicinal products or other substances, taking into account the target group(s) and their corresponding disease status;
- local compatibility and
- toxicity including single dose toxicity, repeated dose toxicity, genotoxicity, carcinogenicity and reproductive and developmental toxicity, depending on the level and nature of exposure to the product.

In the absence of such studies, a justification shall be provided.

This documentation must also be submitted to the consulted regulatory authorities for pharmaceuticals (EMA or national) via the NB as part of a consultation procedure in accordance with Annex IX.5.4 or X.6, as appropriate.

d) MDs containing CMR or endocrine disrupting (ED) substances

(referred to in MDR: Annex I.II. Section 10.4.1.)

Here the justification referred to in Section 10.4.2 of Annex I has to be given (with related documentation). See also chapter 5.3 and 4 of this book (to section 10 of Annex I)[386].

See also EN ISO 22442 series: Medical devices utilizing animal tissues and their derivatives

[386] See SCHEER guidance: Guidelines on the benefit-risk assessment of the presence of phthalates in certain medical devices covering phthalates which are carcinogenic, mutagenic, toxic to reproduction (CMR) or have endocrine-disrupting (ED) properties
https://ec.europa.eu/health/sites/health/files/scientific_committees/scheer/docs/scheer_o_015.pdf

e) Sterility or other defined microbiological condition:

For products placed on the market in a sterile state or with a defined micro-biological condition, a description of the environmental conditions for the relevant manufacturing steps. For products placed on the market in sterile condition, a description of the methods used to package, sterilise and maintain sterility, including validation reports. In the validation report, the bioburden test, pyrogen tests and, if necessary, the examination of sterilising agent residues are also dealt with.

For documentation purposes, special reference is made here to the comprehensive pool of relevant Harmonized Standards, as listed partly in Chapter I.4.4. of this book under "Important Harmonized European Standards for the Medical Devices Directives".

f) Measuring function:

For products placed on the market with a measuring function, a description of the methods used to ensure the accuracy as given in the specifications. See also Annex I.II.15: Products with diagnostic or measurement function. MEDDEV 2.1/5 Medical Devices with a Measuring Function http://ec.europa.eu/DocsRoom/documents/10283/attachments/1/translations may give useful hints.

g) Combinations

For MDs which have to be connected to another MD/products for their intended use, a description of this connection/configuration including proof that the former MD fulfils the general safety and performance requirements with regard to the characteristics specified by the manufacturer when connected to another product.
See also Annex I.II. of the MDR and chapter V.3. in this book.

The conformity assessment modules IX to XI ("Euro-approval") provide for the submission of the technical documentation and its assessment by the NB (partly on a representative basis). Within the framework of market surveillance, the competent authorities may also inspect the TD.

10.2 Technical documentation for IVDs

Source: IVDR, Annex II+III (PMS)

The manufacturer must prepare and keep up to date a technical documentation in accordance with Annexes II and III of the IVDR for the IVDs produced by him, as part of the general manufacturer's obligations in Art. 10.

> This technical documentation must allow an assessment of the conformity of the IVD and of relevant processes with the requirements of the IVDR. It must therefore be well structured and comprehensive as the central document of conformity with the IVDR!

The technical Documentation (TD) has to be presented in a clear, organised, readily searchable and unambiguous manner and shall include in particular the structure and elements listed in Annex II.

The minimum contents of the technical documentation (TD) are specified in Annex II of the IVDR (see survey in fig. 27; the technical documentation for Post-Market Surveillance (PMS) can be found in Annex III (see Chapter XV on PMS in this book).

Minimum content of the Technical Documentation (TD) for IVDs according to Annex II:
1) DEVICE DESCRIPTION AND SPECIFICATION, INCLUDING VARIANTS AND ACCESSORIES
1.1. Device description and specification
(a) product or trade name and a general description of the device including its intended purpose and intended users;
(b) the Basic UDI-DI as referred to in Part C of Annex VI assigned by the manufacturer to the device in question, as soon as identification of this device becomes based on a UDI system, or otherwise a clear identification by means of product code, catalogue number or other unambiguous reference allowing traceability;
Please note: (IVDR: Art. 24. 7: *As part of the technical documentation referred*

to in Annex II, the manufacturer shall keep up-to-date a list of all UDIs that it has assigned).

*(c) the **intended purpose** of the device which may include information on:*

- [387]*what is to be detected and/or measured;*
- *its function such as screening, monitoring, diagnosis or aid to diagnosis, prognosis, prediction, companion diagnostic;*
- *the specific disorder, condition or risk factor of interest that it is intended to detect, define or differentiate;*
- *whether it is automated or not;*
- *whether it is qualitative, semi-quantitative or quantitative;*
- *the type of specimen(s) required;*
- *where applicable, the testing population;*
- *the intended user;*
- *in addition, for companion diagnostics, the relevant target population and the associated medicinal product(s).*

(d) the description of the principle of the assay method or the principles of operation of the instrument;

(e) the rationale for the qualification of the product as a device;

(f) the risk class of the device and the justification for the classification rule(s) applied in accordance with Annex VIII;

(g) the description of the components and where appropriate, the description of the reactive ingredients of relevant components such as antibodies, antigens, nucleic acid primers; and where applicable:

(h) the description of the specimen collection and transport materials provided with the device or descriptions of specifications recommended for use;

(i) for instruments of automated assays: the description of the appropriate assay characteristics or dedicated assays;

(j)for automated assays: a description of the appropriate instrumentation characteristics or dedicated instrumentation;

(k) a description of any software to be used with the device;

(l) a description or complete list of the various configurations/variants of the device that are intended to be made available on the market;

---

[387] Bullets introduced here instead of I, ii, iii, … for better readability

(m) a description of the accessories for a device, other devices and other products that are not devices, which are intended to be used in combination with the device.

1.2. Reference to previous and similar generations of the device

(a) an overview of the previous generation or generations of the device produced by the manufacturer, where such devices exist;

(b) an overview of identified similar devices available on the Union or international markets, where such devices exist.

From the product description, including the intended purpose and the (main) mechanism of action, it should also be possible, to determine everything that is necessary,

- to clarify the <u>qualification</u> of the product as an IVD;
- <u>which general safety and performance requirements acc. to Annex I of IVDR apply</u> to the IVD or not (e.g. chemical/physical/technical specifications incl. possible release of CMR substances or endocrine disruptors). possible release of nanoparticles; microbial status or reprocessibility; drug components; components of human, animal or microbial origin; possible combinations with other IVDs, MDs or other products and interactions with the environment; diagnostic or measuring functions; release/use of ionising/non-ionising radiation; presence of programmable electronic systems or MDSW or software driving or influencing the use of the IVD; presence of an active component; particular mechanical or thermal risks; risks due to release of energy or substances; lay use or POCT);
- <u>which classification rules of Annex VIII apply</u> (incl. sub-rules) software components[388] and their functionality(ies); regarding release of nanoparticles; diagnostic significance; special rules according to Annex VIII.III.7 applicable?)
- <u>whether consultation procedures are to be carried out</u> in the conformity assessment (see chapter XIII.7. in this book);

---

[388] See MDCG 2020-16: Guidance on Classification Rules for in vitro Diagnostic Medical Devices under Regulation (EU) 2017/746 and MDCG 2019-11: Qualification and classification of software - Regulation (EU) 2017/745 and Regulation (EU) 2017/746

With regard to "intended purpose", the following is important:

> *'intended purpose'* means the use for which a device is intended according to the data supplied by the manufacturer on the label, in the instructions for use or in promotional or sales materials or statements or as specified by the manufacturer in the performance evaluation;

When determining the intended purpose, it is also useful to keep in mind the 5 W-questions of the use of the IVD, where applicable, as a guide:

WHO should use the IVD with WHO's specimens, to measure WHAT (which analytes/markers), under WHICH conditions and WHY?

The description of the intended purpose must be consistent and without contradictions or uncertainties throughout all relevant processes:

1) WHO should use/apply the IVD?

- Intended users/applicants (use by health professionals with or without[389] laboratory expertise/ lay people/people with disabilities; specific qualifications or specific characteristics of users required, possibly given by specific inclusion/exclusion criteria? Specific education or training necessary?)

2) On WHOM (on whose/which samples) is the IVD to be applied?

- This refers to the intended target (patient) populations (demographic characteristics such as age, gender, ethnicity, etc.), e.g. adults/children/infants, newborns, pregnant or lactating women; women of childbearing age; very old people; other vulnerable populations; general or specific health-related criteria, populations with specified general health status; with or without (certain) comorbidities or specific medical treatment history [e.g. treatment resistance? Co-medications?]; other aspects); specific indications or contraindications, see below.
- precise medical indications (if applicable)
- any contraindications; further restrictions and warnings, if applicable
- the type of sample(s) required;
- for companion diagnostics, in addition to the relevant target group, the associated medicinal product(s), including the international non-proprietary name (INN) of the associated medicinal product for which the test is a companion test;

3) Under WHICH conditions of use is the IVD to be used?

---

[389] E.g. for POCT point of care testing outside laboratories by health care personnel

e.g.:
- the preanalytics;
- whether it is automatic or not;
- whether it is qualitative, semi-quantitative or quantitative;
- Application environment, application scenarios
- hardware/software platform, operating systems, software environment

4) WHAT is to be detected and/or measured by the IVD (which markers/analytes?);

5) WHY should the IVD be used? (medical purpose)
- its function such as screening, monitoring, diagnosis or diagnostic aid, prognosis, prediction, companion diagnostic in the areas of application specified under 2);
- is intended exclusively or principally to provide information on one or more of the following (see Def. In IVDR, Art. 2 (2), but this must be clearly specified here!
(a) about physiological or pathological processes or conditions,
b) about congenital physical or mental impairments,
c) on the predisposition to a particular health condition or disease,
(d) on the safety and tolerability in po-tenial recipients,
(e) on the likely effects of, or reactions to, treatment; or
(f) to establish or monitor therapeutic interventions.
- Description of test or functional principle, including scientifically unproven mode of action;
- whether it is intended as an initial test, a confirmatory test or a supplementary test;
- If applicable, functional elements (including software) and their contribution to the performance of the IVD;

2. INFORMATION TO BE SUPPLIED BY THE MANUFACTURER
A complete set of
(a) the label or labels on the device and on its packaging, such as single unit packaging, sales packaging, transport packaging in the case of specific management conditions, in the languages accepted in the Member States where the device is envisaged to be sold;

(b) the instructions for use in the languages accepted in the Member States where the device is envisaged to be sold.

Labelling and instructions for use are described very precisely in IVDR: Annex I.III.20 and the sub-items there must be processed exactly, if applicable.

See also EN ISO 20417 (Medical devices — Information to be supplied by the manufacturer) and

EN ISO 15223-1: (Medical devices — Symbols to be used with medical device labels, labelling and information to be supplied — Part 1: General requirements).

See also ISO 18133-series: In vitro diagnostic medical devices — Information supplied by the manufacturer

Product and product-group specific standards may also contain additional and specific elements for label and instructions for use.

Additional information is to be delivered for Class C+D products via the Summary of Safety and Performance (SSP; see IVDR: Art. 29).

3. DESIGN AND MANUFACTURING INFORMATION[390]

3.1. Design information

Information to allow the design stages applied to the device to be understood shall include:

(a) a description of the critical ingredients of the device such as antibodies, antigens, enzymes and nucleic acid primers provided or recommended for use with the device;

(b) for instruments, a description of major subsystems, analytical technology such as operating principles and control mechanisms, dedicated computer hardware and software;

(c) for instruments and software, an overview of the entire system;

(d) for software, a description of the data interpretation methodology, namely the algorithm;

(e) for devices intended for self-testing or near-patient testing, a description of the design aspects that make them suitable for self-testing or near-patient testing.

Relevant information will often come from documentation of the QMS system.

---

[390] To be supplemented by documents from QMS, EN ISO 13485

3.2. Manufacturing information

(a) information to allow the manufacturing processes such as production, assembly, final product testing, and packaging of the finished device to be understood. More detailed information shall be provided for the audit of the quality management system or other applicable conformity assessment procedures;

(b) identification of all sites, including suppliers and sub-contractors, where manufacturing activities are performed.

Relevant information will often come from documentation of the QMS system.

4. GENERAL SAFETY AND PERFORMANCE REQUIREMENTS

The documentation shall contain information for the demonstration of conformity with the general safety and performance requirements set out in Annex I that are applicable to the device taking into account its intended purpose, and shall include a justification, validation and verification of the solutions adopted to meet those requirements. The demonstration of conformity shall also include:

(a) the general safety and performance requirements that apply to the device and an explanation as to why others do not apply;

(b) the method or methods used to demonstrate conformity with each applicable general safety and performance requirement;

(c) the harmonised standards, CS or other solutions applied;

(d) the precise identity of the controlled documents offering evidence of conformity with each harmonised standard, CS or other method applied to demonstrate conformity with the general safety and performance requirements. The information referred to under this point shall incorporate a cross-reference to the location of such evidence within the full technical documentation and, if applicable, the summary technical documentation.

Annex I, Chap. I ("General requirements") will best be worked through with (a precise reference) to the documentation of the performance evaluation (see 10.2.6. below) and chapter VII in this book) and (a precise reference to) the documentation of the risk management system (see point 5 below and chapter 5.1. and Fig. 15 in this book).

For Chapter II of Annex I ("Requirements Regarding Performance, Design and Manufacture"), first look at section 9, which for the IVDR is a central part of performance evaluation with the crucial parameters of analytical and clinical (diagnostic) performance and will be part of the documentation on performance evaluation, see below under point 6 in this chapter of the book.

For the following sections of Annex I. II. it is recommended that these sections and sub-items are systematically walked through using the 4-step procedure in Fig. 16 (**GSPR-Matrix**) or a similar procedure (use a template[391] for each product of your product portfolio!):

1.   Does the GSPR (incl. sub-items) apply/not apply to the IVD (with explanation if NO)?
2.   If a GSPR (incl. sub-items) applies, can compliance with it be demon-strated by presumptions of conformIty In HarmonIsed Standard(s) and/or CS or by reference to alternative solutions (often state of the art standards, mainly from ISO or IEC) with reasoned justification(s)?
3.   Validation and verification with evidence through controlled documents (e.g. test reports, certificates, etc showing compliance with presumptions or justified alternative solutions) as part of the TD;
4.   Concluding assessment for each section of GSPR and sub-item, whether compliance is given by non-applicability or documented evidence under p.3 above;

Chapter III of Annex I ("Requirements Regarding Information supplied with the device") is dealt with by meticulously working through section 20 (IVDR) and the sub-items of this section that apply to the IVD (see also point 2 above).

5. BENEFIT-RISK ANALYSIS AND RISK MANAGEMENT

The documentation shall contain information on:

(a) the benefit-risk analysis referred to in Sections 1 and 8 of Annex I, and

(b) the solutions adopted and the results of the risk management referred to in Section 3 of Annex I.

(see Chapter V.1. of this book on General Safety and Performance Requirements, section Risk Management, Fig. 15 with a survey on the risk management system required, based on a plan for each IVD);

The general documentation of the Risk Management System based on the risk management plan acc. to section 1 and 8 of Annex I will be based on the

---

[391] Make one by analogy to one of the Annexes of MDCG 2021-8: Clinical investigation application/notification documents, which provides a word template for Annex I of the MDR

clinical/diagnostic benefit/risk considerations of the performance evaluation and its documentation (see section X.2.6 below and chapter VII of this book). Apart from this more general part of the risk management, possibly a more detailed description is necessary on the exertion of the minimisation principle "as far as possible"[392] (risk control with 3-step hierarchy of solutions, see Fig. 15) through the sections of Chapter II of Annex I.

6) Review and validation of the IVD
The documentation shall contain the results and critical analyses of all verification and validation tests and/or studies carried out to demonstrate the conformity of the product with this Regulation and in particular the applicable general safety and performance requirements.
This includes:

6.1.) Information on the analytical performance of the IVD
(see also chapter VII and Fig. 19 and Tab. 16 of this book).
Analytical information would encompass:

6.1.1. Specimen type
This Section shall describe the different specimen types that can be analysed, including their stability such as storage, where applicable specimen transport conditions and, with a view to time-critical analysis methods, information on the timeframe between taking the specimen and its analysis and storage conditions such as duration, temperature limits and freeze/thaw cycles.
6.1.2. Analytical performance characteristics
6.1.2.1. Accuracy of measurement
(a) Trueness of measurement This Section shall provide information on the trueness of the measurement procedure and summarise the data in sufficient detail to allow an assessment of the adequacy of the means selected to es-

---

[392] See IVDR: Annex I.I.2. *The requirement in this Annex to reduce risks as far as possible means the reduction of risks as far as possible without adversely affecting the benefit-risk ratio.*

tablish the trueness. Trueness measures apply to both quantitative and qualitative assays only when a certified reference material or certified reference method is available.

(b) Precision of measurement This Section shall describe repeatability and reproducibility studies.

6.1.2.2. Analytical sensitivity

This Section shall include information about the study design and results. It shall provide a description of specimen type and preparation including matrix, analyte levels, and how levels were established. The number of replicates tested at each concentration shall also be provided as well as a description of the calculation used to determine assay sensitivity.

6.1.2.3. Analytical specificity

This Section shall describe interference and cross reactivity studies performed to determine the analytical specificity in the presence of other substances/agents in the specimen. Information shall be provided on the evaluation of potentially interfering and cross-reacting substances or agents on the assay, on the tested substance or agent type and its concentration, specimen type, analyte test concentration, and results. Interferents and cross-reacting substances or agents, which vary greatly depending on the assay type and design, could derive from exogenous or endogenous sources such as:

(a) substances used for patient treatment such as medicinal products;

(b) substances ingested by the patient such as alcohol, foods;

(c) substances added during specimen preparation such as preservatives, stabilisers;

(d) substances encountered in specific specimen types such as haemoglobin, lipids, bilirubin, proteins;

(e) analytes of similar structure such as precursors, metabolites or medical conditions unrelated to the test condition including specimens negative for the assay but positive for a condition that can mimic the test condition.

6.1.2.4. Metrological traceability of calibrator and control material values

6.1.2.5. Measuring range of the assay

This Section shall include information on the measuring range regardless of whether the measuring systems are linear or non-linear, including the limit of detection and describe information on how the range and detection limit *were established. This information shall include a description of specimen type, number of specimens, number of replicates, and specimen preparation including information on the matrix, analyte levels and how levels were established. If applicable, a description of any high dose hook effect and the data supporting the mitigation such as dilution steps shall be added.*

6.1.2.6. Definition of assay cut-off

This Section shall provide a summary of analytical data with a description of the study design including methods for determining the assay cut-off, such as:

(a) the population(s) studied: demographics, selection, inclusion and exclusion criteria, number of individuals included;

(b) method or mode of characterisation of specimens; and

(c) statistical methods such as Receiver Operator Characteristic (ROC) to generate results and if applicable, define grey-zone/equivocal zone.

6.1.3. The analytical performance report referred to in Annex XIII of IVDR

6.2. Information on the clinical performance of the IVD and clinical evidence[393] in the **clinical performance report** as part of the overall **performance evaluation report (PER)**, which includes the performance evaluation plan, the scientific validity, analytical performance and clinical performance reports, the PMPF-plan and the PMPF-evaluation reports, referred to in Annex XIII, together with an assessment and the conclusions of these reports and, where appropriate, annexed documents relating to [clinical] performance studies (clinical performance study plans and reports)[394] and the literature search plans and report(s).

6.3. Stability (excluding specimen stability)

This Section shall describe claimed shelf life, in use stability and shipping stability studies.

6.3.1. Claimed shelf-life

---

[393] See chapter VII of this book; IVDR: Annex XIII and MDCG 2022-2: Guidance on general principles of clinical evidence for In Vitro Diagnostic medical devices (IVDs)
[394] Acc. to IVDR: Annex XIII.A.2 +3 and Annex XIV

This Section shall provide information on stability testing studies to support the shelf life that is claimed for the device. Testing shall be performed on at least three different lots manufactured under conditions that are essentially equivalent to routine production conditions. The three lots do not need to be consecutive. Accelerated studies or extrapolated data from real time data are acceptable for initial shelf life claims but shall be followed up with real time stability studies. Such detailed information shall include:

(a) the study report including the protocol, number of lots, acceptance criteria and testing intervals;

(b) where accelerated studies have been performed in anticipation of the real time studies, the method used for accelerated studies shall be described; (c) the conclusions and claimed shelf life.

6.3.2. In-use stability

This Section shall provide information on in-use stability studies for one lot reflecting actual routine use of the device, regardless of whether real or simulated. This may include open vial stability and/or, for automated instruments, on board stability.

In the case of automated instrumentation, if calibration stability is claimed, supporting data shall be included. Such detailed information shall include:

(a) the study report (including the protocol, acceptance criteria and testing intervals);

(b) the conclusions and claimed in-use stability.

6.3.3. Shipping stability

This Section shall provide information on shipping stability studies for one lot of devices to evaluate the tolerance of devices to the anticipated shipping conditions. Shipping studies may be done under real and/or simulated conditions and shall include variable shipping conditions such as extreme heat and/or cold. Such information shall describe:

(a) the study report (including the protocol, acceptance criteria);

(b) the method used for simulated conditions;

(c) the conclusion and recommended shipping conditions.

6.4. Software verification and validation

The documentation shall contain evidence of the validation of the software, as it is used in the finished device. Such information shall typically include the *summary results of all verification, validation and testing performed in-house and applicable in an actual user environment prior to final release. It shall also address all of the different hardware configurations and, where applicable, operating systems identified in the labelling.*

Specific reference should be made to Section 16 of Annex I (Electronic programmable systems — devices that incorporate electronic programmable systems and software that are devices in themselves) and EN ISO 62304: "Medical device software — Software life-cycle processes").

See also non-legally binding guidance by MDCG:

MDCG 2020-1: Guidance on clinical evaluation (MDR) / Performance evaluation (IVDR) of medical device software

6.5. Additional information required in special cases

(a) In the case of devices placed on the market in a **sterile or defined microbiological condition**, a description of the environmental conditions for the relevant manufacturing steps. In the case of devices placed on the market in a sterile condition, a description of the methods used, including the validation reports, with regard to packaging, sterilisation and maintenance of sterility[395]. The validation report shall also address bioburden testing, pyrogen testing and, if applicable, testing for sterilant residues[396].

(b) In the case of **devices containing tissues, cells and substances of animal, human or microbial origin**, information on the origin of such material and on the conditions in which it was collected. Reference to Section 12 ("Devices incorporating materials of biological origin") of Annex I of IVDR will be useful.

(c) In the case of devices placed on the market with a **measuring function**, a description of the methods used in order to ensure the accuracy as given in the specifications.

See specifically Annex I.II.14: Devices with a measuring function.

MEDDEV 2.1/5 Medical Devices with a Measuring Function

---

[395] See extensive list of harmonized European standards to deal with sterility and hygienic issues of IVDs and MDs, as partly referenced in chapter 1.4.4. of this book.
[396] See e.g. EN ISO 10993-7: Biological evaluation of medical devices — Part 7: Ethylene oxide sterilization residuals

http://ec.europa.eu/DocsRoom/documents/10283/attachments/1/translations may give useful hints.

(d) If the device is to be **connected to other equipment** in order to operate as intended, a description of the resulting **combination** including proof that it conforms to the general safety and performance requirements set out in Annex I when connected to any such equipment having regard to the characteristics specified by the manufacturer.
See also Annex I.II. of the IVDR and chapter V.5. in this book.

The conformity assessment modules IX to XI provide for the submission of the technical documentation and its assessment by the NB (partly on a representative basis). Within the framework of market surveillance, the competent authorities may also inspect the TD.

Chapter 11. Classification

Annex VIII of both Regulations

Before manufacturers can place a medical device or IVD on the market for the first time or put it into service, they must carry out a suitable conformity assessment, unless the product falls under a "special route" (see Chapter XII.2 or XIII.2 in this book). The conformity assessment ("European Pre-market Approval") is modularly structured according to the principles of the Global Approach; the permissible module combinations are to be selected according to the class of the medical device or IVD: the higher the class, the more stringent the approval procedure.

In addition to conformity assessment, classification also plays a role in the procedures for clinical investigations of MDs (see chapter VIII in this book), in reporting in the context of post-market surveillance (see chapter XV in this book), in custom-made devices (class III implants), in transition periods for the attachment of UDI carriers (see chapter I.6. in this book), etc. Sub-classes of Class I may be important for the date of application of the MDR[397]! It is also important now for transition periods for IVDs acc. to Amendment Regulation (EU) 2022/112.

Please note that the classification of MD/IVD under the new MDR/IVDR must be explicitly carried out under the QMS which is mandatory for the manufacturer! This means greater care in procedures, resources, qualifications and documentation.

---

[397] See chapter 1.6 in this book

234

XI.1 Classification of Medical Devices According to MDR

Sources (legally binding):

- MDR: Article 51 and Annex VIII
- Decisions of European Court of Justice (ECJ)
- Changes to the relevant legal situation regarding classification may result from:
  - Corrigenda or amendments to the MDR (specifically to Art. 51 and Annex VIII)
  - COM implementing acts pursuant to Article 51 of the MDR
  - New Judgments of the European Court of Justice
  - Formal decisions of the Competent Authorities (CA) or Courts of Member States[398] (also in case of disputes between manufacturer and NB)

Non-legally binding interpretative guidance on classification:

MDCG 2021-24: Guidance on classification of medical devices
MDCG 2019-11: Qualification and classification of software in Regulation (EU) 2017/745 and Regulation (EU) 2017/746; this makes the previous
MANUAL on borderline and classification: aims only at MDD and AIMDD (and IVDD); the "individual decisions" of the stakeholders on certain MD types listed here so far are only of limited use for the purposes of the MDR. Always perform a gap analysis towards MDR! According to reports, the MANUAL will not be systematically transferred to the MDR; new "decisions" of the Manual will in any case refer then to the MDR (and possibly to the IVDR);
- there may be national Interpretive guidelines for the classification of MDs issued by Member States;
- Other interpretation aids from stakeholder organisations[399]

The more than half a million different medical devices on the European market represent a very heterogeneous group of products, from walking aids, medical device apps to devices for magnetic resonance imaging (MRI)

---

[398] These may be overruled by the ECJ
[399] These are legally the "weakest" of the non-legally binding guidelines

and catheter-based heart valve implants (TAVI[400]). To be able to define adequate approval procedures for the individual medical device groups and the associated risks, these are divided into classes (note: medical devices and IVDs each have their own classification).

In MDR, medical devices are classified acc. to **Art. 51** into **classes I, IIa, IIb and III** in accordance with the rules of **Annex VIII**, taking into account their **intended purpose** and the associated risks; Class III represents the highest risk class.

Class I can still be differentiated into 4 subgroups[401]:

Class I: (non-sterile; without measuring function; no reusable surgical instrument of class I)
Class Is: sterile class I medical device
Class Im: Class I medical device with measuring function
Class Ir: reusable surgical instrument of Class I.

For **performing a classification under the MDR**, the following must be observed (see Fig. 28):

- assure you have the **current version** of legally binding and interpretative, non-legally binding sources, for classification at hand
- Check the **intended purpose** of the MD[402]
- The **definitions** in Annex VIII.I.,
- the **7 implementing rules** ("meta-rules") in Annex VIII.II. and above all,
- the **22 rules** including sub-rules in Annex VIII.III. The rules are again structured according to **invasiveness** of MD[403] (non-invasive - invasive), presence of an energy source (**active** MD, incl. software, – non-active MD) and according to **special rules**. All rules including sub-rules are to be checked and documented during classification; the strictest rule or

---

[400] TAVI: transcatheter aortic valve implantation
[401] Necessary for the purposes of conformity assessment, see chapter XII.6.4. in this book, as Im, Ir and Is will need a NB under the MDR
[402] See chapter 10.I. in this book; your intended purpose should be precise enough to decide on applicability of each classification rule/sub-rule
[403] See the further differentiation and escalation to higher classes for different kinds of invasiveness in Fig. 28

sub-rule resulting in the highest classification shall apply and determine the class of the MD.

Tip: get hold of a template for a matrix of the 22 rules incl. the sub-rules as lines, to clearly and reproducibly check applicability/non-applicability of a rule or sub-rule to your MD with appropriate reasoning and to what risk class that will lead in the columns. The highest risk class achieved will count!

Examples of important changes/additions of the MDR to the classification of Directive 93/42/EEC - while largely maintaining its' current structure - include:

IVF/ART[404]: All non-invasive devices consisting of a substance or a mixture of substances intended to be used in vitro in direct contact with human cells, tissues or organs taken from the human body or used in vitro with human embryos before their implantation or administration into the body are classified as class III[405].

All implantable devices and long-term surgically invasive devices are classified as class III[406], if they e.g.
- are active implantable devices or their accessories,
- are breast implants or surgical meshes,
- are total or partial joint replacements, with the exception of ancillary components such as screws, wedges, plates and instruments; or
- are spinal disc replacement implants or are implantable devices that come into contact with the spinal column, with the exception of components such as screws, wedges, plates and instruments.

---

[404] IVF: in-vitro fertilization; ART: Artificial reproduction technology
[405] See MDR, Annex VIII, Rule 3, 2nd para
[406] See MDR, Annex VIII, Rule 8; please note that there are a lot of other, additional device groups mentioned under this rule!

Software[407]:

Software intended to provide information which is used to take decisions with diagnosis or therapeutic purposes is classified as class IIa, except if such decisions have an impact that may cause:

- death or an irreversible deterioration of a person's state of health, in which case it is in class III; or
- a serious deterioration of a person's state of health or a surgical intervention, in which case it is classified as class IIb.

Software intended to monitor physiological processes is classified as class IIa, except if it is intended for monitoring of vital physiological parameters, where the nature of variations of those parameters is such that it could result in immediate danger to the patient, in which case it is classified as class IIb. All other software is classified in Class I.

All devices manufactured **utilising tissues or cells of human or animal origin**, or their derivatives, which are non- viable or rendered non-viable, are classified as class III, unless such devices are manufactured utilising tissues or cells of animal origin, or their derivatives, which are non-viable or rendered non-viable and are devices intended to come into contact with intact skin only.

Nanomaterials:

All devices incorporating or consisting of nanomaterial are classified as[408]:

- class III if they present a high or medium potential for internal exposure;
- class IIb if they present a low potential for internal exposure; and
- class IIa if they present a negligible potential for internal exposure.

Devices that are composed of **substances or of combinations of substances**[409] that are intended to be introduced into the human body via a body

---

[407] See MDR, Annex VIII, Rule 11; see specifically also: MDCG 2019-11: Qualification and classification of software - Regulation (EU) 2017/745 and Regulation (EU) 2017/746 and MDCG 2021-24: Guidance on classification of medical devices
[408] See MDR, Annex VIII, Rule 19; details to be expected in guidance
[409] See MDR, Annex VIII, Rule 21

orifice or applied to the skin and that are absorbed by or locally dispersed in the human body are classified as:

- class III if they, or their products of metabolism, are systemically absorbed by the human body in order to achieve the intended purpose;
- class III if they achieve their intended purpose in the stomach or lower gastrointestinal tract and they, or their products of metabolism, are systemically absorbed by the human body;
- class IIa if they are applied to the skin or if they are applied in the nasal or oral cavity as far as the pharynx, and achieve their intended purpose on those cavities; and
- class IIb in all other cases.

Active therapeutic devices with an integrated or incorporated diagnostic function[410] which significantly determines the patient management by the device, such as closed loop systems or automated external defibrillators, are classified as class III.

---

[410] See MDR, Annex VIII, Rule 22

239

Classification rules MDR, Annex VIII

Fig. 28 MDR Annex VIII Classification Rules Survey

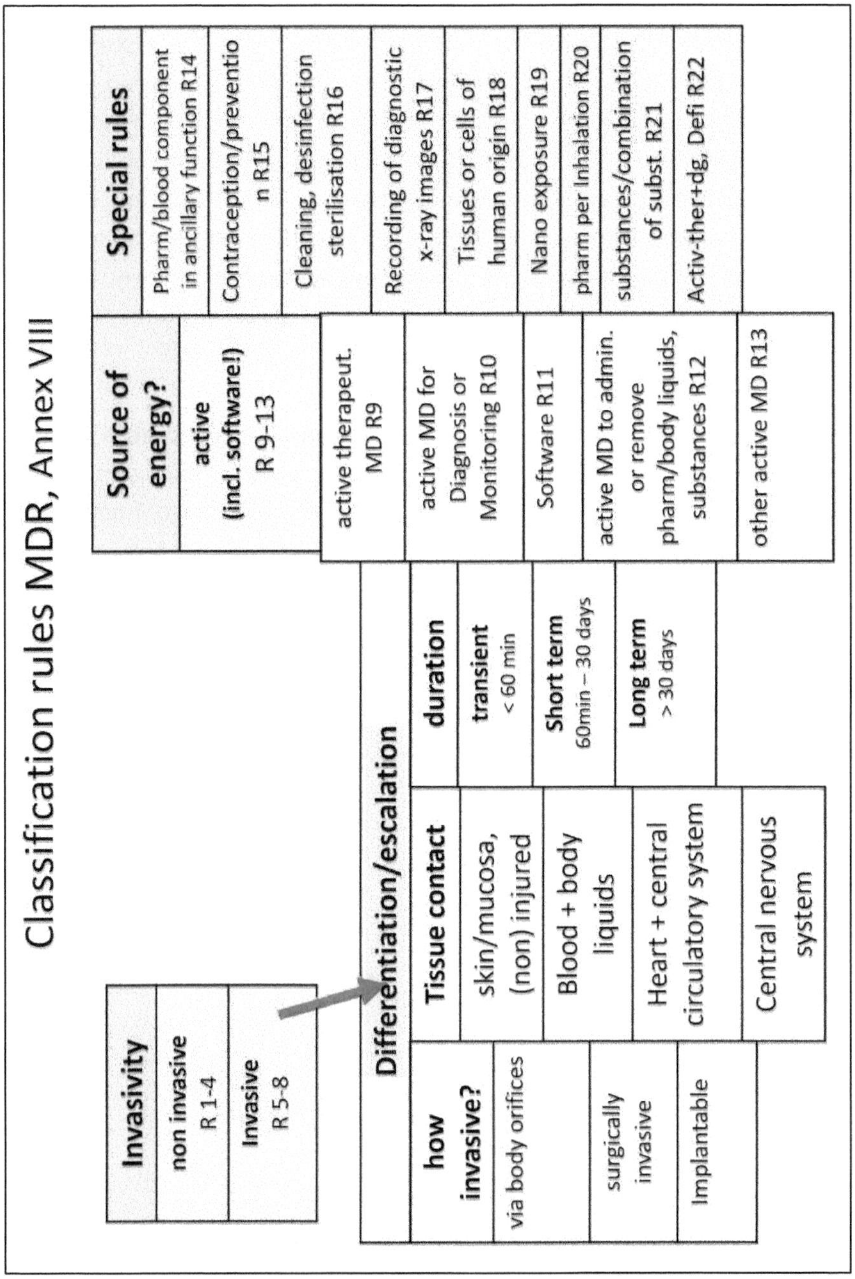

Invasivity

Invasivity	
non invasive	R 1-4
Invasive	R 5-8

Special rules

Special rules
Pharm/blood component in ancillary function R14
Contraception/prevention R15
Cleaning, desinfection sterilisation R16
Recording of diagnostic x-ray images R17
Tissues or cells of human origin R18
Nano exposure R19
pharm per Inhalation R20
substances/combination of subst. R21
Activ-ther+dg, Defi R22

Source of energy?

active (incl. software!) R 9-13
active therapeut. MD R9
active MD for Diagnosis or Monitoring R10
Software R11
active MD to admin. or remove pharm/body liquids, substances R12
other active MD R13

Differentiation/escalation

duration	Tissue contact	how invasive?
transient < 60 min	skin/mucosa, (non) injured	via body orifices
Short term 60min – 30 days	Blood + body liquids	surgically invasive
Long term > 30 days	Heart + central circulatory system	Implantable
	Central nervous system	

XI.2 Classification of In Vitro Diagnostics According to IVDR

Sources (legally binding):
- IVDR: Article 47 and Annex VIII
- Decisions of European Court of Justice (ECJ)
- (National): Formal decisions of the Competent Authorities (CA) or Courts of Member States (also in case of disputes between manufacturer and NB)
- Changes to the relevant legal situation regarding classification may result from:
  - Corrigenda or amendments to the IVDR (specifically to Art. 47 and Annex VIII)
  - COM implementing acts pursuant to Article 47 of the IVDR
  - New Judgments of the European Court of Justice
  - Changes to national formal interpretations by formal decisions of CA or national courts

Non-legally binding interpretative guidance on classification:
- MDCG 2020-16 rev1: Guidance on Classification Rules for in vitro Diagnostic Medical Devices under Regulation (EU) 2017/746
- MDCG 2019-11: Qualification and classification of software in Regulation (EU) 2017/745 and Regulation (EU) 2017/746;
- there may be national Interpretive guidelines for the classification of IVDs issued by Member States;
- Other interpretation aids from stakeholder organisations[411]

In vitro diagnostics also represent a very heterogeneous product group, from established culture media, blood collection tubes to IVDs for cancer diagnostics, to infection markers, blood group reagents that are crucial for the safety of blood and tissue products or IVDs for medical genetic diagnostics and companion diagnostics used e.g. in cancer management. Particular attention must also be paid to self-tests for lay persons or Point of Care Testing (POCT). In order to define adequate approval procedures for the individual IVD

---

[411] These are legally the "weakest" of the non-legally binding guidelines

groups and the associated risks, these are divided into classes (note: medical devices and IVDs each have their own classification!).

IVDs are classified in the IVDR into **classes A, B, C, D**, taking into account their intended purpose and the associated risks. This classification scheme largely (but with some changes!) follows the relevant IVD classification guideline of GHTF/IMDRF[412], where Class D represents the highest risk class.

The classification of IVDs takes into account the manufacturer's intended purpose for its IVD and the risks associated with it, in accordance with Annex VIII of the IVDR.

An essential element of Annex VIII are the **7 classification rules** (in VIII.II.; many with sub-rules!) for classification.

The application of the rules is governed by **10 implementing rules** in VIII.I.

The rationale of the new classification based on the GHTF/IMDRF guideline lies in the consideration of individual and public health risk in the various classes (Tab. 20)

Tab. 20 GHTF/IMDRF and IVDR: Rationale for Risk Classification of IVDs

Class	Risk constellation
A	Low Individual Risk and Low Public Health Risk
B	Moderate Individual Risk and/or Low Public Health Risk
C	High Individual Risk and/or Moderate Public Health Risk
D	High Individual Risk and High Public Health Risk

[412] Acc to: Principles of IVD Medical Devices Classification
SG1 Final Document GHTF/SG1/N045:2008 http://www.imdrf.org/docs/ghtf/final/sg1/pro-cedural-docs/ghtf-sg1-n045-2008-principles-ivd-medical-devices-classification-080219.pdf

Tab. 21 IVDR, Annex VIII: Survey of IVD-Classification, Examples

Class	Rule(s)	Examples of IVD groups or markers for[413]
D	1+2	• ABO-, Rhesus-, Kell-, Kidd-, Duffy-system[414]; • Transmissible agent in blood (components), cells, tissues or organs or their derivatives[415]; • Transmissible agent that causes life threatening disease[416]; • Infectious load of a life-threatening disease[417]
C[418]	2-4	• IVDs for blood grouping or tissue typing other than those in Class D[419]; • Sexually transmitted agent; • infectious agent in cerebrospinal fluid or blood; • companion diagnostics; monitoring of levels of medicinal products[420]; • human genetic testing; • screening, diagnosis or staging of cancer; • screening for congenital disorders in embryo, fetus or new-born babies; pre-natal screening of women for immune status; • disease staging; management of patients suffering from life-threatening disease or condition;
B[421]	4, 6, 7	• IVDs for self-testing for pregnancy, fertility testing and cholesterol level; urine tests for glucose, erythrocytes, leukocytes and bacteria; • Controls without assigned quantitative or qualitative value; • B=fallback Class!
A	5	• Specimen receptacles; • instruments specifically for IVD-procedures • accessories without critical characteristics, general culture media and biological stains, buffer and washing solutions, etc., intended by the MF to make them suitable for IVD-procedures relating to a specific examination

---

[413] For details see always IVDR: Annex VIII.2.; items displayed here may be highly abbreviated!

[414] ABO system [A (ABO1), B (ABO2), AB (ABO3)]; — Rhesus system [RH1 (D), RHW1, RH2 (C), RH3 (E), RH4 (c), RH5 (e)]; — Kell system [Kel1 (K)]; — Kidd system [JK1 (Jka), JK2 (Jkb)]; — Duffy system [FY1 (Fya), FY2 (Fyb)];

For **performing a classification under the IVDR**, the following must be observed (see Tab. 21):
assure you have the **current version** of legally binding and interpretative, non-legally binding, sources for classification at hand![422]

---

[415] detection of the presence of, or exposure to, a transmissible agent in blood, blood components, cells, tissues or organs, or in any of their derivatives, in order to assess their suitability for transfusion, transplantation or cell administration;

[416] detection of the presence of, or exposure to, a transmissible agent that causes a life-threatening disease with a high or suspected high risk of propagation;

[417] determining the infectious load of a life-threatening disease where monitoring is critical in the process of patient management.

[418] IVDR: Annex VIII, Rule 3: Devices are classified as class C if they are intended:
(a) for detecting the presence of, or exposure to, a sexually transmitted agent;
(b) for detecting the presence in cerebrospinal fluid or blood of an infectious agent without a high or suspected high risk of propagation;
(c) for detecting the presence of an infectious agent, if there is a significant risk that an erroneous result would cause death or severe disability to the individual, fetus or embryo being tested, or to the individual's offspring;
(d) for pre-natal screening of women in order to determine their immune status towards transmissible agents;
(e) for determining infective disease status or immune status, where there is a risk that an erroneous result would lead to a patient management decision resulting in a life-threatening situation for the patient or for the patient's offspring;
(f) to be used as companion diagnostics;
(g) to be used for disease staging, where there is a risk that an erroneous result would lead to a patient management decision resulting in a life-threatening situation for the patient or for the patient's offspring;
(h) to be used in screening, diagnosis, or staging of cancer;
(i) for human genetic testing;
(j) for monitoring of levels of medicinal products, substances or biological components, when there is a risk that an erroneous result will lead to a patient management decision resulting in a life-threatening situation for the patient or for the patient's offspring;
(k) for management of patients suffering from a life-threatening disease or condition;
(l) for screening for congenital disorders in the embryo or fetus;
(m) for screening for congenital disorders in new-born babies where failure to detect and treat such disorders could lead to life-threatening situations or severe disabilities.

[419] Devices intended to be used for blood grouping, or tissue typing to ensure the immunological compatibility of blood, blood components, cells, tissue or organs that are intended for transfusion or transplantation or cell administration, are classified as class C, except ... *(Class D)*

[420] Also called drug monitoring

[421] Class B is fallback class: IVDR: Annex VIII, Rule 6: Devices not covered by the above-mentioned classification rules are classified as class B.

[422] This will have to be continuously monitored in the change management under your QMS!

- Check the **intended purpose** of the IVD[423]
- the **10 implementing rules** ("meta-rules") in Annex VIII.I. and above all,
- the **7 rules** including sub-rules in Annex VIII.II. All rules including sub-rules are to be checked and documented during classification; the strictest rule or sub-rule resulting in the highest classification shall apply and determine the class of the MD.

Tip: get hold of a template for a matrix of the 7 rules incl. the sub-rules as lines, to clearly and reproducibly check applicability/non-applicability of a rule or sub-rule to your IVD (under consideration of the implementing rules, with appropriate reasoning) and to what risk class that will lead, depicted in the columns. The highest risk class achieved will count!

In IVDR, we now have a **risk-rule-based classification system** that can react adequately in a rule based mode to new developments in the IVD sector; the previous system had been list-based (list A and List B of Directive 98/79/EC) and therefore relatively inflexible.

---

[423] See chapter 10.2. in this book; your intended purpose should be precise enough to decide on applicability of each classification rule/sub-rule

Chapter 12. Conformity Assessment of MDs

("European Premarket Approval" for Medical Devices)

How can I legally place medical devices on the market or put them into service in the EU/EEA according to MDR?

How can my MD legally reach the user in EU/EEA following the MDR?

Before first placing on the market or in the case of MDs which are not placed on the market, before they are (first) put into service, MDs (and their manufacturers – Art. 10) must prove their conformity with the requirements of the MDR. After various preliminary clarifications, this evidence of conformity is to be provided and documented within the framework of defined conformity assessment procedures ("European Premarket Approval") under the principles of the Global Approach[424]. The main route of conformity assessment will lead to **CE marking of conformity**[425]. In order to find the correct way to the market/user, some preliminary considerations are necessary:

12.1. The Preliminary Clarifications for MDs

- Does the **product fall under the MDR**? (see chapter II.1 in this book)
- Is the product to be CE marked or is it covered by a **special route without CE marking** (see below under XII.2)?
- Does the product also fall under **other EU legislation**[426], especially those requiring CE marking and/or a EU declaration of conformity? (these regulations would then also have to be fulfilled if necessary!
- The **classification** of the product according to Annex VIII of the MDR (see chapter 11.1.).

Please note: In addition to the Global Approach Procedure, which leads (in a positive case) to CE marking, there are also strictly defined '**special routes**' for certain conditions, which guarantee access to the market or the user for certain MDs without CE marking:

---

[424] See chapter 1.2.3. in this book
[425] Unless "Special Routes" apply, see chapter 12.2 below
[426] Think eg. of Machinery Directive 2006/42/EC; Radio Equipment Directive 2014/53/EU; Low Voltage Directive 2014/35/EU; have a look also to Blue Guide 2016 of COM, specifically list of legislation on page 14, to check for possible applicability

12.2. Checks for "Special Routes" (Outside CE-marking)

- **Investigational MDs** (MDR: Chapter VI; see chapter VIII in this book[427]);
- **In-house production** (MDR: Art. 5 (5); production in/for health care facilities of the EU): under strictly defined cumulative conditions, only the general safety and performance requirements of Annex I may apply here![428]
- **Custom Made Devices**[429] (CMD; MDR: Art. 2 No. 3; Art. 52 (8); Annex XIII): for Class III implants, NB according to Annex IX.I. (QMS) or Annex XI.A (Production Quality Assurance) required! For CMDs, a statement in accordance with Annex XIII.1 and a documentation in accordance with Annex XIII.2 must be prepared[430].
- **Systems and procedure packs**[431] (MDR: Art. 2 (11)+(10); Art. 22) In addition to MDs with CE marking according to MDR, products of other legislations[432] may now also be part of a (medically meaningful) system or procedure pack. Where such systems or procedure packs are sterilised for placing on the market, a conformity assessment procedure with NB

---

[427] Usually clinical investigations (except PMCF-studies) are performed before conformity assessment and CE-marking

[428] Member States may issue stricter rules!

[429] *'custom-made device'* means any device specifically made in accordance with a written prescription of any person authorized by national law by virtue of that person's professional qualifications which gives, under that person's responsibility, specific design characteristics, and is intended for the sole use of a particular patient exclusively to meet their individual conditions and needs.

However, mass-produced devices which need to be adapted to meet the specific requirements of any professional user and devices which are mass-produced by means of industrial manufacturing processes in accordance with the written prescriptions of any authorized person shall not be considered to be custom-made devices;

E.g. Dental bridges and crowns for individual patients are usually considered custom made devices; in future 3-D printing may be considered here.

[430] See also MDCG 2021-3: Questions and Answers on Custom-Made Devices

[431] *'procedure pack'* means a combination of products packaged together and placed on the market with the purpose of being used for a specific medical purpose;

'system' means a combination of products, either packaged together or not, which are intended to be inter- connected or combined to achieve a specific medical purpose;

[432] Eg. IVDs; Personal protective equipment; biocides; medicinal products: these non-MD components have to comply with their resp. legislation.

> in accordance with Annex IX or XI.A concerning the sterilisation aspects must be carried out.
> - **Exemptions**[433] (MDR: Art. 59) granted by Member States and/or COM
> - (**Exhibitions, fairs** and similar events: = not to be considered making available on the market!)

If a 'special route' is not applicable, the route must be taken via the main road to market in the EU/EEA:

12.3. The Modular Conformity Assessment Procedure for CE Marking (Overview)

In accordance with the principles of the Global Approach, the main route of "European Premarket Approval" leads via a modular conformity assessment procedure to CE marking, as a sign of conformity with the applicable European regulations (overview: Path to CE marking in Fig. 29).

The modules suitable for a MD (= Annexes IX - XI or parts thereof; partly in conjunction with Annexes II+III = Technical Documentation) are determined by the class of the MD and usually give the manufacturer certain options of choice. **Art. 52 of MDR** tells the manufacturer which modules will be eligible for which class of MD. The higher the risk class, the more stringent the modules become. Conformity assessment for low-risk products (= Class I, but without Im, Is or Ir) is carried out by the manufacturer himself, without a NB[434]; from a medium risk on (i.e. from Class Im, Is or Ir and higher classes) the involvement of a suitable Notified Bodies (NB) is obligatory.

---

[433] Similar to Emergency Use Authorizations and Humanitarian Device Exemption Program of FDA

[434] these MFs will anyhow be under market surveillance by MS

Fig. 29 MDR/IVDR: Path to CE Marking of Conformity

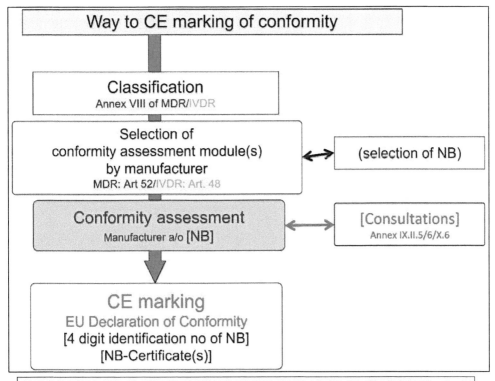

12.4. How to Find a Suitable Notified Body for my MD/MDs?

The conformity assessment of the MD from class Is, Im, Ir and higher is carried out with the help of Notified Bodies (NB). The following considerations apply to the individual product as well as to the product portfolio as a whole, since as a rule one usually wants to carry out conformity assessments with a notified body within "already established" procedures[435].

If both MD and IVD are in the portfolio, one should pay attention to whether the NB - if so desired - can operate both product portfolios!

---

[435] Please note: As a general rule, a lead auditor of the NB shall neither lead nor attend audits for more than three consecutive years in respect of the same manufacturer (Annex IX.I.3.6).

The NB must be selected on the basis of the notification scope of the notified bodies, which is the range of qualification assigned to the NB by the Designating National Authority. This scope is determined for MDR on the basis of 3 main criteria and the associated multidimensional codes (so-called "NBOG codes") specified in the Commission Implementing Regulation (EU) 2017/2185 concerning the scope of the designation of a Notified Body within the framework of MDR and IVDR[436]:

- **Product type** and its MDA codes (for active MD) or MDN codes (for non-active MD), each further subdivided into implantable or non-implantable MDs[437] and further on.
- **Horizontal competence codes** referring to
  - **Specific Characteristics** of MD (MDS codes), e.g. with medicinal substances; with tissues; sterile; with software; with nanomaterials, etc]
  - **Technologies or processes used** (MDT codes), e.g. metal processing; plastic processing; biotechnology; clean room conditions; electronic components; etc.

Annexes IX - XI of the MDR which the manufacturer could apply.

---

[436] COMMISSION IMPLEMENTING REGULATION (EU) 2017/2185 of 23 November 2017 on the list of codes and corresponding types of devices for the purpose of specifying the scope of the designation as notified bodies in the field of medical devices under Regulation (EU) 2017/745 of the European Parliament and of the Council and in vitro diagnostic medical devices under Regulation (EU) 2017/746 of the European Parliament and of the Council: https://eur-lex.europa.eu/legal-content/EN/TXT/?uri=CELEX:32017R2185 . For MDR the codes are in Annex I of this legal act. See also MDCG 2019-14: Explanatory note on MDR codes

[437] Strictly speaking the division for **active devices** is:
Active implantable devices; Active non-implantable devices for imaging, monitoring and/or diagnosis; and: Active non-implantable therapeutic devices and general active non-implantable devices; versus for **non-active devices**:
Non-active implants and long term surgically invasive devices; and: Non-active non-implantable devices;

Fig. 30 MDR Codes for NBs

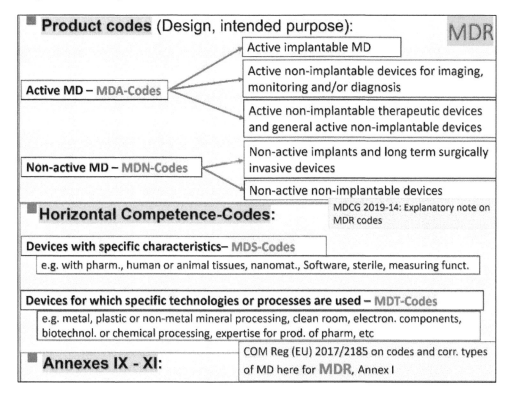

Search procedure for NBs, portfolio search: You will determine the product type codes for your current product portfolio and its extensions planned in the short or medium term. Then look at the horizontal competence codes found in the current and planned portfolio. Finally, you determine which Annex (usually Annex IX is selected) or which Annexes you need or want to use after classifying your products. Codes and Annex(es) lead you to the "possible" NBs!

Search method for NBs, single product search: You determine the product type code again and check which product code and which horizontal competence codes apply to your product. Finally, check which Annex(es) match(es) your product classification and which one(s) you want to choose. Codes and Annex(es) lead you to the "possible" NBs!

The search for a suitable NB should be performed via the **NANDO-Information System[438] of EU**. After clicking to legislation and then selecting Regulation (EU) 2017/745 for MDR the currently designated NBs for the MDR will be displayed. You may filter then with the help of 3 pull down menus for product types, horizontal competence codes valid for your MDs and Annexes chosen for conformity assessment.

Alternatively you may directly inspect the competence profile of a "desired NB" by a direct click on it in the NANDO.

If your desired NB is still in the process of designation, you as the manufacturer should make sure in good time in writing! that your "planned" NB has already submitted its application for designation according to the MDR/IVDR[439] and which product types, horizontal codes and Annexes have been applied for. Perform a gap analysis of your product portfolio and develop a plan B (other NB or additional NB?) if necessary[440].

In addition to these absolutely essential criteria of suitability of a NB within MDR for a product or product portfolio in question, which are to be determined on the basis of the codes and the desired annex(es), **other criteria** usually also play a role:

- The **language requirements** for documents or audits that the NB requires (may be determined by the NB's Member State or the NB itself);
- The **NB's time (acute and long-term) resources** for handling the conformity assessment of the product or product portfolio;
- The **costs of conformity assessment** and the necessary audits;
- **Experience with the NB**;
- Does the NB participate in the **MDSAP** (Medical Device Single Audit Program)[441]?

---

[438] Nando (New Approach Notified and Designated Organisations) Information System https://ec.europa.eu/growth/tools-databases/nando/

[439] Which was possible from 26 November 2017

[440] See state of play of designations under COM homepage: https://ec.europa.eu/docsroom/documents/32026

[441] E.g. www.imdrf.org or https://www.fda.gov/medical-devices/cdrh-international-programs/medical-device-single-audit-program-mdsap

For certain types of high-risk MDs, the NB must also conduct supplementary **consultation procedures** with certain authorities (e.g. authorities for medicinal products; tissue authorities; competent authorities for MD), EU reference laboratories (for IVDs) or with expert panels, which all prepare scientific opinions to be observed in the conformity assessment by the NB. The positive completion of conformity assessment modules is documented by **certificates of the Notified Bodies** according to Annex XII of the MDR.

12.5. Overview: Conformity Assessment According to Annex IX-XI

The conformity assessment modules of MDR include in particular the following annexes (incl. subchapters) of the MDR:

- Annex IX (QMS and assessment of technical documentation)
- Annex X (Type examination)
- Annex XI (Product conformity testing)

In most conformity assessment modules the assessment of the technical documentation of **Annex II and III** (see chapter X in this book; assessment is partly on a representative basis) plays an important role.

12.5.1. Overview: Annex IX

based on a **QMS and the assessment of the technical documentation, TD** (see Fig. 31 and 32):

Choice for classes IIa - III, also for Im, Is, Ir: here restricted to QMS and administrative regulations and to the respective special aspects. Class III implantable Custom Made Devices now also require Annex IX.I. or Annex XI.A. Annex IX includes 3 chapters:

- **QMS (Chapter I: Sections 1-3)** (see Fig. 31):
  - Section 1: Overview QMS
  - Section 2: QMS application, implementation, documentation, Audits, QMS changes
  - Section 3: Surveillance assessment for Classes IIa - III
- **Assessment of the TD (Chap. II; Sections 4-6)** (see Fig.32):

- Section 4: General assessment of TD for Class III and for IIb implants[442] for each product; for other IIb and for IIa on a representative basis[443];
- Section 5: Consultation procedures, where applicable;
- Section 6: Batch Control of blood components, if applicable;

- **Administrative provisions (Chap. III: Sections 7-8,** keeping documents demonstrating conformity available for competent authorities for at least 10 years, for implants at least 15 years after the last product has been placed on the market; Member State regulates the availability of documents in the event of bankruptcy by the manufacturer.

---

[442] With some exemptions, which may be later changed by implementing Acts of the COM

[443] See also MDCG 2019-13: Guidance on sampling of devices for the assessment of the technical documentation

Fig. 31 MDR: Annex IX QMS and TD Assessment Overview

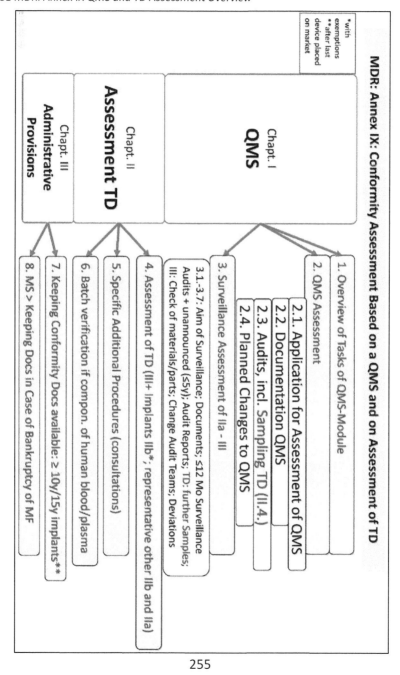

255

Fig. 32 MDR: Annex IX TD Assessment Overview

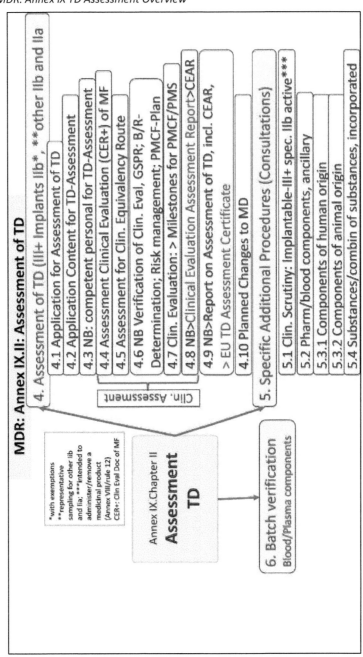

12.5.2. Overview: Annex X

Conformity assessment based on **EU type examination**

Applicable for Classes III and IIb in combination with Annex XI (Part A or B);
Annex X includes 7 Sections:

1. procedure overview;
2. application
3. evaluation by NB
4. EU type-examination certificate;
5. type modifications;
6. specific additional procedures (consultation procedures, reference to IX.II.5.)
7. administrative provisions (keeping documents of conformity available for competent authorities)

12.5.3. Overview Annex XI

Conformity assessment based on **product conformity verification**
Choice between:
Part A: production quality assurance (XI.A);
Part B: product testing (XI.B)
For Classes III and IIb in combination with Annex X; for Class IIa in combination with TD according to Annex II+III; for Class I only in special cases (Part A is option for Im, Is or Ir, limited to special aspects). Custom Made Class III implants now also require Annex XI.A or Annex IX.I

It should be noted that the **European conformity assessment is not a single event, but accompanies the life cycle of the MD**. NB certificates are only valid for a limited period (max. 5 years) and must be renewed in due time; manufacturers can expect at least annual audits of their QMS and unannounced audits at least all 5y (life-cycle conformity assessment). NBs are also involved in the flow of relevant PMS and vigilance reports of manufacturers. The NB and its consultation partners also intervene in the event of planned changes.

Finally, above all, there is **Market Surveillance by Competent Authorities - CA**; see Chapter VII.3 of both Regulations.

257

12.6. Conformity Assessment for MDs of Classes III - I according to MDR: Art. 52

MD must first be assigned to Class I (I, Im, Is, Ir), IIa, IIb or III in accordance with Annex VIII. Depending on the class, the manufacturer has different options of conformity assessment modules for his MD, codified in Art. 52.

The following schemes are not applicable to custom made devices (CMD) and investigational devices.

Whereas consultation procedures (reference to Annex IX.II.5+6) are theoretically possible for all classes of MD's [MDR: Art. 52 (8) – (11)], a "realistic" view reveals, that this will only be applicable to Class III and some Class IIb MDs.

12.6.1. Class III:

(Fig. 33): According to Art. 52 (3), manufacturers of MDs of Class III are subject to conformity assessment in accordance with

- **Annex IX, I-III** (QMS and assessment of TD)
  + consultations (Annex IX.II.5+6), if applicable,

OR

- **Annex X** (EU type examination)
  + consultations, if applicable (ref. to Annex IX.II.5)

AND

- **Annex XI** (product conformity verification):

  o **Part XI.A** [Production Quality Assurance]
    + Consultations (if applicable)

  OR

  o **Part XI.B** [Product Verification]
    + Consultations (if applicable)

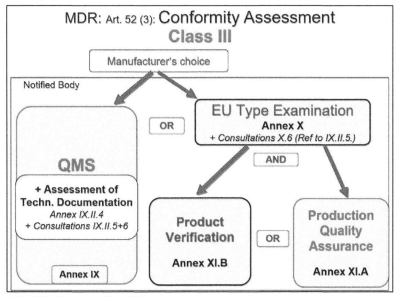

Fig. 33 MDR: Overview Class III Conformity Assessment

259

12.6.2. Class IIb:

(Fig. 34); According to MDR: Art. 52 (4) + (5) manufacturers of MDs of Class IIb are subject to conformity assessment in accordance with

- **Annex IX, I-III** (QMS and assessment of TD)

  + assessment of TD for IIb implants[444]

  + representative assessment of TD of other IIb-MDs[445] (≥1/generic MD-group)

  + consultations (IX.II.5+6), if applicable,

OR

- **Annex X** (EU type examination)

  + consultations (ref to IX.II.5), if applicable,

  AND

- **Annex XI** (product conformity verification):

  - **Part XI.A** [Production Quality Assurance]
    OR
  - **Part XI.B** [Product Verification]
    + consultations, if applicable

---

[444] With exceptions: sutures, staples, plates, pins, wires, clips, screws, wedges, etc; the list of exceptions may be amended by the COM by delegated acts; see Art. 52 (4) and (5).

[445] Additional sampling for TD-assessments will be taken in the surveillance at each audit by the NB; see MDCG 2019-13: Guidance on sampling of devices for the assessment of the technical documentation

Fig. 34 MDR: Overview Class IIb Conformity Assessment

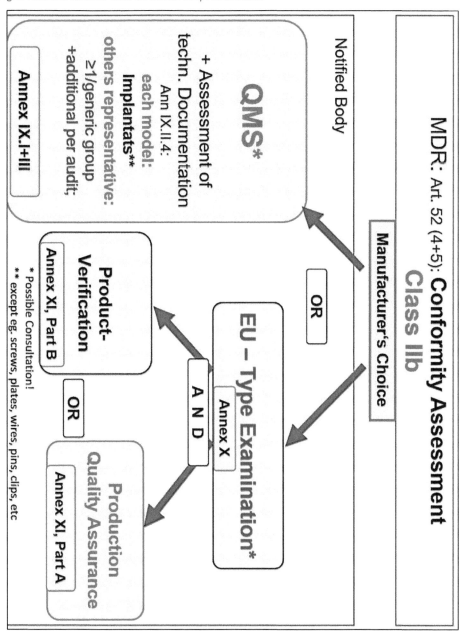

12.6.3. Class IIa:

(Fig. 35); according to Art. 52 (6), manufacturers of MDs of Class IIa are subject to a conformity assessment with

- **Annex IX, I+III (**QMS)
  + **representative assessment of TDs**[446] (≥1/MD-category)
  + **consultations** (IX.II.5+6), if applicable,

OR

- **Annex II+III** (Technical Documentation; manufacturer!)

  AND

- **Annex XI** (product conformity verification):

  o **Part XI.A** [Production Quality Assurance], Section 10
  + representative assessment of TD (≥ 1/MD category)[447]
  OR
  o **Part XI.B** [Product Verification], Section 18

---

[446] Additional sampling for TD-assessments will be taken at each audit of NB
[447] Further samples of TD are taken per MD-category during surveillance audits by NBs; see MDCG 2019-13: Guidance on sampling of devices for the assessment of the technical documentation

Fig. 35 MDR: Overview Class IIa Conformity Assessment

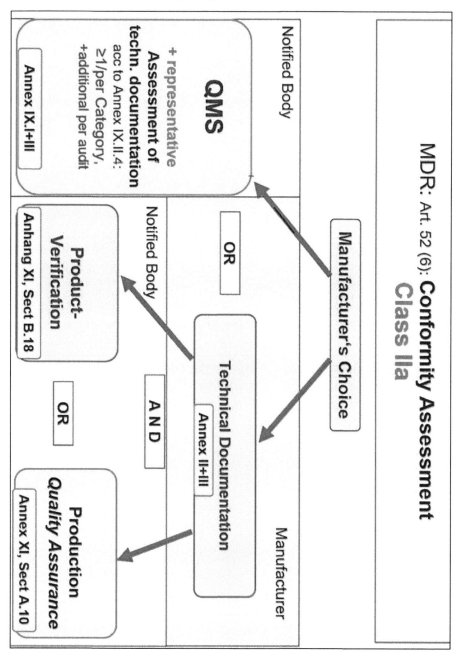

12.6.4. Class I:

(Fig. 36);[448] in accordance with Article 52 (7), Manufacturers of MDs of Class I follow the following procedures: **The manufacturer draws up**

- **the Technical Documentation acc to Annex II + III** and the
- **EU Declaration of Conformity acc to Art. 19/Annex IV**

Additionally, for Is, Im, Ir, the manufacturer follows these procedures for certain Class I-MDs, each restricted to the specific aspects below:

- **Annex IX Chapt. I + III**

OR

- **Annex XI Part A**

Restricted to these aspects:

➔ **Is:** For **Class I-MDs placed on the market in sterile condition** (in relation to aspects relating to the manufacture, securing and maintenance of sterile conditions);

➔ **Im:** For **class I-MD with measuring function** (related to aspects related to the conformity of the MD with the metrological requirements);

➔ **Ir:** For **reusable surgical instruments as Class I-MD** (in relation to aspects related to reuse, in particular cleaning, disinfection, sterilisation, maintenance and functional testing and the associated instructions for use)

---

[448] See also MDCG 2019-15 rev1: Guidance notes for manufacturers of class I medical devices

Fig. 36 MDR: Overview Class I Conformity Assessment

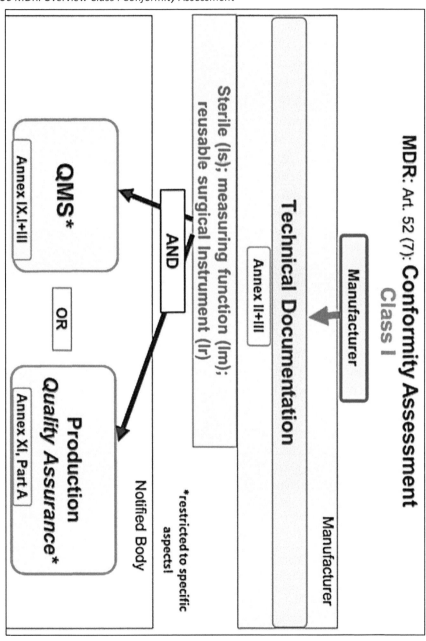

12.7. Consultation Procedures

According to Art. 52 (9)-(11) of the MDR, certain types of MD also require consultation with an authority or an expert panel (in addition to the intervention of a NB), whose scientific opinions must then be observed by the NB; in some cases the NB is even formally bound to this scientific opinion, i.e. it may not issue a certificate if the opinion in the consultation expertise is negative! In principle, consultations are possible for every class, but in fact they only take place for the highest risk classes! The consultations are described in Annex IX.5+6 (Tab. 22) and are referenced in Annex X.6:

Tab. 22 MDR: Overview of Consultation Procedures for Conformity Assessment

- **Annex IX.5.1: Assessment of NB's clinical assessment (CEAR and manufacturer's clinical documentation (CER, CEV plan; PMCF plan; PMCF evaluation reports]) by an EU panel of experts on Class III implants and certain Class IIb active MDs**[449];
  (21d advance notice; 60d from transmission of documents by COM))
- **Annex IX.5.2: MD with ancillary medicinal substance** (also from human blood or plasma) by a national authority for medicinal products or EMA; binding![450]
  (210d pV[451] ; changes: 60d pV)
- **Annex IX.5.3.1: MD containing non-viable tissues, cells or derivatives of human origin**[452] by the tissue authority of a Member State; binding!
  (120d pV; changes: 60d pV)
- **Annex IX.5.3.2: MD from/with tissue, cells of animal origin or their derivatives:** the procedure under Regulation (EU) 722/2012 (to prevent possible transmission of TSEs[453]) with consultation of Member States authorities will

---

[449] See details of this rather complicated procedure in MDR: Art. 54 and Annex IX.II.5.1 + MDCG 2019-3 rev.1: Interpretation of article 54(2)b

[450] See EMA-Guidance: European Medicines Agency recommendation on the procedural aspects and dossier requirements for the consultation of the European Medicines Agency by a notified body on an ancillary medicinal substance or an ancillary human blood derivative incorporated in a medical device or active implantable medical device https://www.ema.europa.eu/en/documents/regulatory-procedural-guideline/ema-recommendation-procedural-aspects-dossier-requirements-consultation-ema-notified-body-ancillary_en.pdf

[451] pV: post validation of documents

[452] These might be MDs (derivatives) acc to Art. 1. 6 (g), 2nd half-sentence or ancillary components acc to Art. 1.10, 1st subpara

[453] TSE: Transmissible Spongiform Encephalopathies; like CJD, vCJD or BSE, Scrapie; see: https://eur-lex.europa.eu/LexUriServ/LexUriServ.do?uri=OJ:L:2012:212:0003:0012:EN:PDF

be continued under MDR;
(12 Weeks: if without EDQM[454] certificate; 4 weeks if with EDQM certificate)

- **Annex IX.5.4: MDs composed of substances or combinations of substances absorbed by or locally dispersed in the human body;** consultation with an authority for medicinal products (national or EMA); (150d pV)[455]

- **Annex IX.6 (Batch verification**; also Annex XI.A.8. and Annex XI.B.16) describes the procedure for MD with a supporting medicinal substance derived from human blood or plasma as an integral part, where the manufacturer provides the NB with an official certificate from a state or OMCL[456] laboratory on the release of the batch of human blood or plasma derivative used in this product for each batch release.

12.8. After Successful Conformity Assessment (Classes I-III)

If successful, the NB issues

- **certificate(s)** (valid for a maximum of 5 years) and allow the manufacturer to affix its

- **NB's 4-digit identification number**, as a sign of successful "European Premarket Approval"

The manufacturer can then issue the

- **EU Declaration of Conformity** on that basis (for class A non-sterile on the manufacturer's own responsibility without the NB certificate!) in the required languages of the MS where the placing on the market is being planned and

- affix the **CE marking** (with the NB's 4 digit identification number (if a NB has been involved),

- and then start marketing[457]. Furthermore, if not already done before,

- the **registration obligations** and the **UDI obligations** according to the specific schedule (see chapter 1.6 and 4 of this book) must be fulfilled.

---

[454] EDQM - European Directorate for the Quality of Medicines & HealthCare

[455] See EMA Guidance on the interfaces MDs and pharmaceuticals: https://www.ema.europa.eu/en/human-regulatory/overview/medical-devices

[456] Official Medicines Control Laboratory (OMCL) is an official laboratory for the investigation and independent quality control of medicinal products and other similarly regulated substances

[457] Unless other legislations, which also apply to that product still have to be fulfilled

Conformity assessment is not a singular event: after successful certification it also includes regular, usually annual, and also unannounced **audits by the NB** (at least once in 5 years) and timely insight of the NB into current PMS and vigilance reports of the manufacturer. Furthermore, **planned changes** to the product, its intended purpose or the QMS are subject to evaluation by the notified body, which, depending on the scope and relevance of the planned change[458], may lead to a **supplement to the EU certificate** on the assessment of the TD or the QMS or the EU type examination certificate, or to **a new conformity assessment** in accordance with Art. 52 of the MDR. A new consultation with consulted authorities may also be necessary.

In the case of **implantable Class III** MDs and **certain active Class IIb MDs**, an additional control mechanism (**Mechanism for Scrutiny**) by MS, COM or expert panel is also foreseen in accordance with Art. 55 (market surveillance immediately after certification).

Note: The general manufacturer obligations with the life cycle processes (above all QMS, risk management, clinical evaluation with PMCF, PMS and vigilance, registration obligations, traceability, communication with competent authorities and other stakeholders) remain in force in the further course (see Chapter 3.1. in this book)!

---

[458] See NBOG document NBOG BPG 2014-3: Guidance for manufacturers and Notified Bodies on reporting of Design Changes and Changes of the Quality System: https://www.nbog.eu/nbog-documents/ :"It is recommended that manufacturers contact and discuss with their Notified Body about any questions related to the substantial or not substantial characteristic of the change in order to get a common understanding."

Chapter 13. Conformity Assessment of IVDs

("European Premarket Approval" of IVDs)

How can I legally place IVDs on the market or put them into service in the EU/EEA according to IVDR?

How can my IVD legally reach the user in EU/EEA following the IVDR?

Before (first) placing on the market or in the case of IVDs which are not placed on the market, before they are (first) put into service, IVDs (and their manufacturers – Art. 10) must prove their conformity with the requirements of the IVDR. After various preliminary clarifications, this evidence for compliance is to be provided and documented within defined conformity assessment procedures ("European Premarket Approval"): The main route of conformity assessment[459] will lead to CE marking of conformity[460].

Please note: Contrary to the IVDD, now the large majority of IVDs under the IVDR will need a NB for conformity assessment![461]

In order to find the correct way to the market/user, some preliminary considerations are however necessary:

13.1. Preliminary Clarifications for IVDs

- Does the **product fall under the IVDR?** (see chapter 2.2 in this book)
- Is the **product to be CE marked** or is it covered by a **"special route"** without CE marking (see below under XIII.2)?
- Does the product also fall under **other EU legislation[462]**, especially those requiring CE marking and/or an EU declaration of conformity? (these legislations would then also have to be fulfilled if necessary!
- The **classification** of the product according to Annex VIII of the IVDR (see chapter 11.2.).

---

[459] See chapter 1.3 in this book

[460] Unless "Special Routes" apply, see chapter 12.2 below

[461] Acc. to MedTech Europe, the rate of IVDs where a NB is needed will raise from 8% to 78%

[462] Think e.g. of Machinery Directive 2006/42/EC; Radio Equipment Directive 2014/53/EU; Low Voltage Directive 2014/35/EU; have a look also to Blue Guide 2016 of COM, specifically list of legislation on page 14, to check for possible applicability. A new version of the Blue Guide of the COM has been announced.

Please note: In addition to the Global Approach Procedure, which leads (in a positive case) to CE marking, there are also strictly defined **"special routes"** for certain conditions, which guarantee access to the market or the user for certain IVDs without CE marking:

13.2. Checks for "Special Routes" (Outside CE-marking)

- **IVDs for performance study** (IVDR: Chapter VI; see chapter VIII in this book);
- **In-house production** (IVDR: Art. 5 (5); production in/for health care facilities of the EU): under strictly defined cumulative conditions, only the essential safety and performance requirements of Annex I may apply here![463]. Please note postponed transition time limits under the Amendment Regulation (EU) 2022/112.
- **Exemptions**[464] (IVDR: Art. 54) granted by Member States and/or COM
- (**Exhibitions, fairs** and similar events: = not making available on the market!)

If a special route is not applicable, the route must be taken via

13.3. The Modular Conformity Assessment Procedure for CE Marking (Overview)

In accordance with the principles of the Global Approach, the main route of "European Premarket Approval" leads via a modular conformity assessment procedure to the CE marking, as a sign of conformity with the applicable European legislation (overview: Path to CE marking in Fig. 37).

The modules suitable for an IVD (= Annexes IX - XI or parts thereof; partly in conjunction with Annexes II+III = Technical Documentation) are determined by the class of the IVD and usually give the manufacturer certain options of choice. **Art. 48 of IVDR** tells the manufacturer which modules will be eligible for which class of the IVD. The higher the risk class, the more stringent the modules become. Conformity assessment for low-risk products (= Class A, non sterile) is carried out by the manufacturer himself, without a NB; from a

---

[463] Please note: Member States may issue stricter rules!

[464] Similar to Emergency Use Authorizations (EUA) or Humanitarian Device Exemption Program of FDA

medium risk on (i.e. from Class A sterile and higher classes) the involvement of a suitable Notified Body[465] (NB) is obligatory.

Fig. 37 MDR/IVDR: Path to CE Marking of Conformity

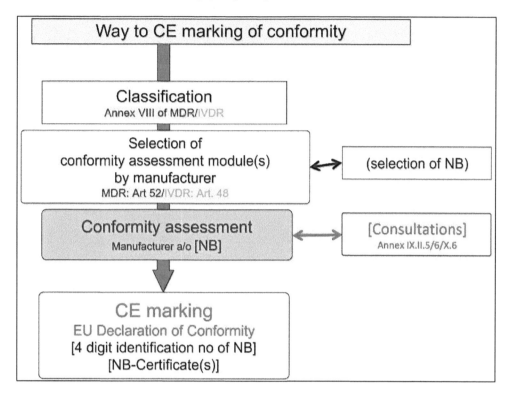

13.4. How do I Find a Suitable Notified Body for my IVD(s)?

Conformity assessment of IVDs of Class A sterile and higher is carried out with the help of notified bodies under IVDR. The following consideration is to be applied to the individual product as well as to the product portfolio as a

---

[465] Combinations of modules (Annexes IX – XI; e.g. Annex X + XI for Class D or C) may be provided by the same or by different suitable NBs eligible by the manufacturer.

whole, since one usually wants to carry out conformity assessments with a notified body within "established routine procedures" if possible[466].

If both MDs and IVDs are in your portfolio, you should pay attention to whether the NB - if so desired - can serve both product portfolios!

The NB must be selected on the basis of the notification scope of the notified bodies. This is determined on the basis of **3 main criteria** (Product type; Horizontal Competence Codes; Annexes) and the associated multidimensional codes, specified in the Commission Implementing Regulation (EU)

Fig. 38 IVDR: NB codes

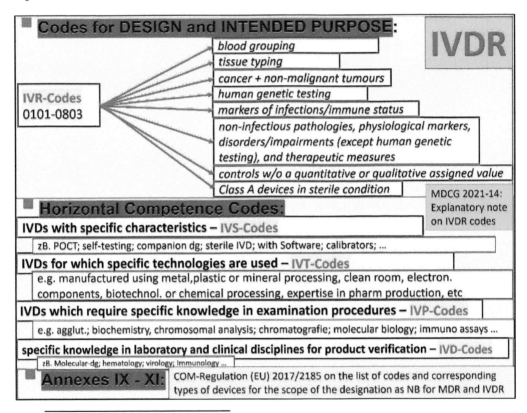

[466] But please note: As a general rule, a lead auditor of the NB shall neither lead nor attend audits for more than three consecutive years in respect of the same manufacturer (Annex IX.I.3.6).

272

2017/2185 concerning the scope of the designation of a Notified Body within the MDR and IVDR[467] (Fig. 38):

- **Product type** and its IVR codes (IVR codes relating to design and intended purpose, divided into 8 subgroups) For IVDs, these codes currently range from products for blood group determination (from IVR 0101) to sterile products of Class A (up to IVR 0803).
- **Horizontal competence codes**, which refer to
  - **S**pecific characteristics of IVDs (IVS codes)[468],
  - **T**echnologies used (IVT codes)[469],
  - IVDs which require specific knowledge in examination **P**rocedures for the purpose of product verification (IVP codes)[470]; and
  - IVDs which require specific knowledge in laboratory and clinical **D**isciplines for the purpose of product verification (IVD codes)[471].
- **Annexes IX - XI** or sub-modules which the NB can serve.

<u>Search procedure NB, portfolio search:</u> You will determine the **product type** codes for your current product portfolio and its possible extensions planned in the short or medium term. Then look at the **horizontal codes** found in the current and planned portfolio. Finally, you define which **Annex(es)** (usually Annex IX) you need or want to use after the classification of your products. Codes and Annex(es) lead you to the NBs in question!

<u>Search method NB, single product search:</u> You determine the product type code again and check which horizontal codes apply to your product. Finally, check which Annex(es) match(es) your product classification and which one(s) you want to choose from. Codes and Annex(es) lead you to the NBs in question!

---

[467] https://eur-lex.europa.eu/legal-content/EN/TXT/?uri=CELEX:32017R2185 . Please look also at MDCG 2021-14: Explanatory note on IVDR codes

[468] Eg. Near patient testing; self-testing; companion diagnostics; software etc.

[469] Eg. Biotechnology, electronic components; metal or plastic processing; etc

[470] Biochemistry, immunoassays; radioactivity; chromosomal analysis

[471] Eg. Bacteriology; clinical chemistry; molecular biology; immunology; etc

If your desired NB is not yet listed in NANDO, you as the manufacturer should make sure in good time in writing! that your "planned" NB has already been designated as a NB under the IVDR or at least has already submitted its application for designation according to the MDR/IVDR and which product types, horizontal product codes and Annexes have been applied for[472]. Perform a gap analysis of your (also planned) product portfolio and develop a plan B (additional NB?) if necessary.

The search for suitable NBs for IVDR should be carried out via the NANDO system of the EU[473].

In addition to these 3 absolutely essential criteria of the basic suitability of a NB for a product or product portfolio, which are to be selected on the basis of the codes and the desired annexes, **other criteria** usually also play a role:

- The **language requirements** for documents or audits that the NB requires (may be determined by the NB's Member State or the NB itself);
- The **NB's time resources** (short and medium-term) for handling the conformity assessment of the product or product portfolio;
- The **costs** of conformity assessment and the necessary audits;
- **Experience** with the NB;
- Does the NB participate in the **MDSAP** (Medical Device Single Audit Program)[474]?

13.5. Overview: Conformity Assessment According to Annexes IX-XI

The conformity assessment modules of IVDR include in particular the following annexes (incl. subchapters) of the IVDR:

- Annex IX (QMS and assessment of technical documentation)

---

[472] This has been possible from 26 November 2017; See state of play of designations under COM homepage: https://ec.europa.eu/docsroom/documents/40341

[473] NANDO: check for desired legislation IVDR 2017/746: https://ec.europa.eu/growth/tools-databases/nando/index.cfm?fuseaction=directive.notifiedbody&dir_id=35

[474] E.g. www.imdrf.org or https://www.fda.gov/medical-devices/cdrh-international-programs/medical-device-single-audit-program-mdsap

- Annex X (Type examination)
- Annex XI (Production Quality Assurance)

In most conformity assessment modules the assessment of the technical documentation of **Annex II and III** (partly on a representative basis) plays an important role.

13.5.1. Overview: Annex IX

based on a **QMS and the assessment of the technical documentation (TD; partly representative)**

Choice for classes B – D; also, for Class A sterile: here restricted to sterility aspects.

Annex IX includes 3 chapters:

- **QMS (Chapter I: Sections 1-3)** (see Fig. 39):
  - Section 1: Overview QMS
  - Section 2: QMS assessment: application, implementation, documentation, Audits, QMS changes
  - Section 3: Surveillance assessment for Classes (B – D)

- **Assessment of the TD (Chapt. II; Sections 4+5)** (see Fig. 40):
  - Section 4: Assessment of TD for Class B, C, D and batch verification of Class D
  - Section 5: Assessment of TD for specific types of IVDs:
    - Self-testing, POCT[475];
    - Companion diagnostics;
- **Administrative provisions (Chapt. III: Sections 6-7,** keeping documents demonstrating conformity available for competent authorities for at least 10 years after the last product has been placed on the market; Member State regulates the availability of documents in the event of bankruptcy of the manufacturer).

---

[475] POCT: Point of Care Testing = near-patient testing

Fig. 39 IVDR: Annex IX QMS+TD Overview

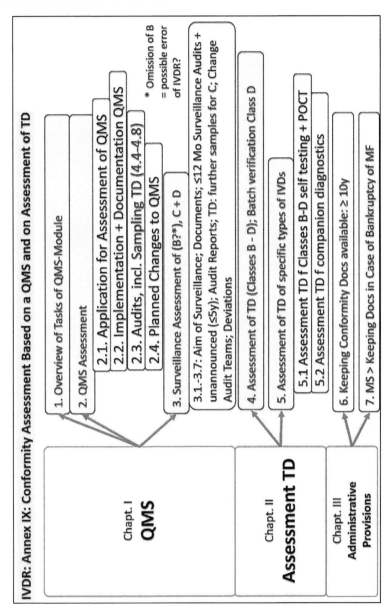

IVDR: Annex IX: Conformity Assessment Based on a QMS and on Assessment of TD

Chapt. I
QMS

1. Overview of Tasks of QMS-Module

2. QMS Assessment

2.1. Application for Assessment of QMS

2.2. Implementation + Documentation QMS

2.3. Audits, incl. Sampling TD (4.4.4.8)

2.4. Planned Changes to QMS

3. Surveillance Assessment of (B?*), C + D

3.1.-3.7: Aim of Surveillance; Documents; ≤12 Mo Surveillance Audits + unannounced (≤5y); Audit Reports; TD: further samples for C; Change Audit Teams; Deviations

* Omission of B = possible error of IVDR?

Chapt. II
Assessment TD

4. Assessment of TD (Classes B - D); Batch verification Class D

5. Assessment of TD of specific types of IVDs

5.1 Assessment TD f Classes B-D self testing + POCT

5.2 Assessment TD f companion diagnostics

Chapt. III
Administrative Provisions

6. Keeping Conformity Docs available: ≥ 10y

7. MS > Keeping Docs in Case of Bankruptcy of MF

Fig. 40 IVDR: Annex IX TD, Overview

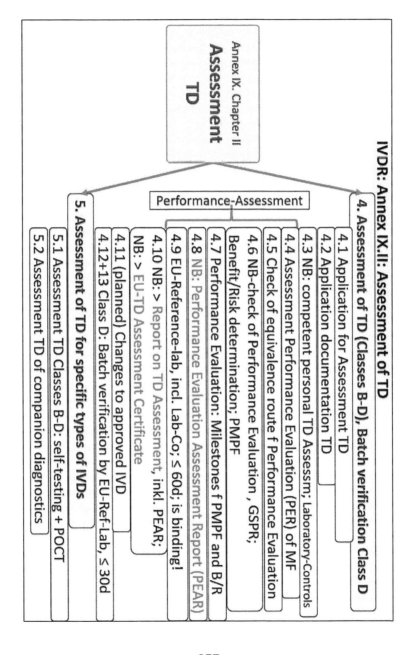

IVDR: Annex IX.II: Assessment of TD

Annex IX. Chapter II
**Assessment
TD**

Performance-Assessment

4. Assessment of TD (Classes B-D), Batch verification Class D

4.1 Application for Assessment TD

4.2 Application documentation TD

4.3 NB: competent personal TD Assessm; Laboratory-Controls

4.4 Assessment Performance Evaluation (PER) of MF

4.5 Check of equivalence route f Performance Evaluation

4.6 NB-check of Performance Evaluation , GSPR;

Benefit/Risk determination; PMPF

4.7 Performance Evaluation: Milestones f PMPF and B/R

4.8 NB: Performance Evaluation Assessment Report (PEAR)

4.9 EU-Reference-lab, incl. Lab-Co; ≤ 60d; is binding!

4.10 NB: > Report on TD Assessment, inkl. PEAR;

NB: > EU-TD Assessment Certificate

4.11 (planned) Changes to approved IVD

4.12+13 Class D: Batch verification by EU-Ref-Lab, ≤ 30d

5. Assessment of TD for specific types of IVDs

5.1 Assessment TD Classes B-D: self-testing + POCT

5.2 Assessment TD of companion diagnostics

13.5.2. Overview: Annex X

Conformity assessment based on **EU type examination**

Applicable for Classes D and C in combination with Annex XI;

Annex X includes 7 Sections:

1. Procedure overview;
2. Application
3. Assessment by NB [incl. consultation with EU reference lab + poss. Expert panel for Class D (X.3.j) and of medicinal product Authority for Companion diagnostics (X.3.k)];
4. EU type-examination certificate;
5. Changes to the type;
6. Administrative provisions (keeping documents of conformity available for competent authorities)

13.5.3. Overview Annex XI

Conformity assessment based on **Production Quality Assurance**

For Classes D and C in combination with Annex X; for Class A sterile: limited to sterility aspects.

It should be noted that the **conformity assessment is not a single event** but accompanies the life cycle of the IVD. NB certificates are only valid for a limited period (max. 5 years) and must be renewed in due time; manufacturers can expect at least annual audits of their QMS and unannounced audits[476] (life-cycle conformity assessment). NBs are also involved in the flow of relevant PMS and vigilance reports of Class C and D manufacturers. The NB and its consultation partners also intervene in the event of planned (significant) changes.

Finally, above all, **market supervision by the competent authorities** (Competent Authorities - CA; Chapter VII.3 of both Regulations) will have a close look at IVDs and their manufacturers, esp. in case of non-conformities.

---

[476] At least once in 5 years

13.6. Overview: The Conformity Assessment Procedures for Classes D to A

The options for conformity assessment modules for IVDs (with the exception of products for performance studies) corresponding to certain Classes are set out in Article 48 of the IVDR.

13.6.1. IVD Conformity Assessment Class D:

(Fig. 41) According to IVDR: Art. 48 (3) to (6) Class D IVD manufacturers are subject to a conformity assessment following:

- **Annex IX, Chapt. I (QMS) + III (administrative provisions)** AND
- **Annex IX, Chapt. II (Assessment of technical documentation),** section 5 only applied in specific cases[477]

> **+ scientific opinion of EU Ref lab acc to IX.II.4.9**[478]
> **+ scientific opinion of expert panel**[479]
> **+ Batch testing of each batch by EU Ref lab, NB and Manufacturer (≤ 30d)**[480]
> **+ Annex IX.II.5.1** for **IVD for self-testing and POCT**[481];

---

[477] Section 5 is only applied as follows: 5.1 for IVD for self-testing and POCT (Point of Care Testing = near-patient tests); 5.2 for companion diagnostics;

[478] For Class D IVDs for which one or more EU ref labs have been designated: the notified body shall request an EU reference laboratory, where designated in accordance with Article 100, to verify the performance claimed by the manufacturer and the compliance of the device with the CS, where available, or with other solutions chosen by the manufacturer to ensure a level of safety and performance that is at least equivalent. The verification shall include laboratory tests by the EU reference laboratory as referred to in Article 48(5).

[479] If no CS is available for this (kind of) product, and this is the 1st certification for that type of device, the NB consults the expert panel (Art. 106 of MDR!). See also MDCG 2021-22: Clarification on "first certification for that type of device" and corresponding procedures to be followed by notified bodies, in context of the consultation of the expert panel referred to in Article 48(6) of Regulation (EU) 2017/746

[480] Batch testing is described in Annex IX.4.12+13 resp. Annex XI.5.1+2

[481] POCT: Point of Care Testing; 5.1. is concerned with the specific assessment of TD, especially as regards these specific user groups and situations, as well as their (possibly limited) qualifications and interpretation potentials, which may also be covered by specific study results.

+ Annex IX.II.5.2 for **companion diagnostics** (with consultation of a competent authority for medicinal products [nat. or EMA][482])

OR

- **Annex X (EU Type-examination)**

  + scientific opinion of EU Ref lab acc to X.3.(j)
  + scientific opinion of expert panel acc to X.3.(j)
  + consultation of a competent authority for medicinal products [nat. or EMA]) **for companion diagnostics** acc to X.3.(k)

  AND

- **Annex XI (Production Quality Assurance)**

  + Batch testing of each batch by EU Ref lab, NB and Manufacturer (≤ 30d)[483]

---

[482] https://www.ema.europa.eu/en/human-regulatory/overview/medical-devices#companion-diagnostics-('in-vitro-diagnostics')-section

[483] Batch testing is described in Annex IX.4.12+13 resp. Annex XI.5.1+2

Fig. 41 IVDR: Class D Overview Conformity Assessment

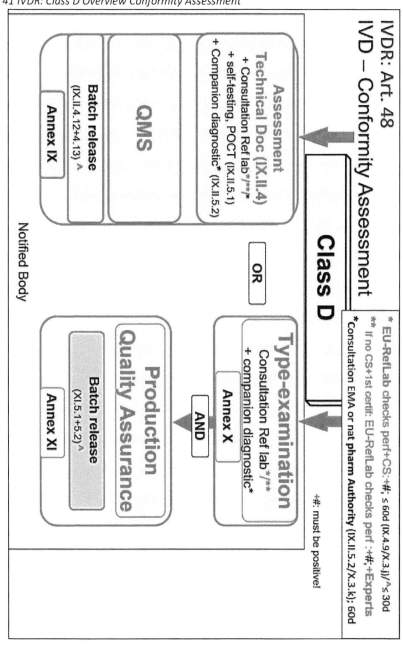

IVDR: Art. 48
IVD – Conformity Assessment

Class D

Notified Body

Assessment
Technical Doc (IX.II.4)
+ Consultation Ref lab*/**
+ self-testing, POCT (IX.II.5.1)
+ Companion diagnostic* (IX.II.5.2)

QMS

Batch release
(IX.II.4.12+4.13) ^

OR

Type-examination
Consultation Ref lab*/**
+ companion diagnostic*

Annex X

AND

Production
Quality Assurance

Batch release
(XI.5.1+5.2) ^

Annex XI

* EU-RefLab checks perf+CS: +#; ≤ 60d (IX.4.9/X.3.i)/^≤ 30d
** If no CS+1st certif: EU-RefLab checks perf : +#, +Experts
* Consultation EMA or nat **pharm Authority** (IX.II.5.2/X.3.k); 60d

+#: must be positive!

281

13.6.2. IVD Conformity Assessment Class C:

(Fig. 42); According to IVDR: Art. 48 (7) and (8), Manufacturers of IVDs of Class C are subject to a conformity assessment of

- **Annex IX, Chapt. I (QMS)[484] + III (administrative provisions)**

AND

- **Annex IX, Chapt. II (Assessment of TD)** acc to Annex IX.II.4. for at least 1 representative example per generic device group[485]

> **+ Annex IX.II.5.1 for IVD for self-testing and POCT[486];**
> **+ Annex IX.II.4.1-4.8. + Annex IX.II.5.2 for companion diagnostics** (with consultation of Authority for medicinal products, nat. or EMA[487])

OR

- **Annex X (EU-Type-examination)**
  + Annex X.3.k for companion diagnostics (with consultation of Authority for medicinal products, nat. or EMA[488])

AND

- **Annex XI (Production Quality Assurance)** without section 5[489]

---

[484] During surveillance audits the NB has to draw further samples of TD per generic device group and assess the TD acc to Annex IX.II.4.4.-4.8; see also Annex VII.4.5.2.a) 4th indent
[485] For sampling, see MDCG 2019-13: Guidance on sampling of devices for the assessment of the technical documentation
[486] POCT: Point of Care Testing = near patient testing
[487] https://www.ema.europa.eu/en/human-regulatory/overview/medical-devices#companion-diagnostics-('in-vitro-diagnostics')-section
[488] For EMA guidance, see footnote above!
[489] Section 5 is only applicable to Class D (Batch testing by EU Ref lab)

Fig. 42 IVDR: Class C Conformity Assessment Overview

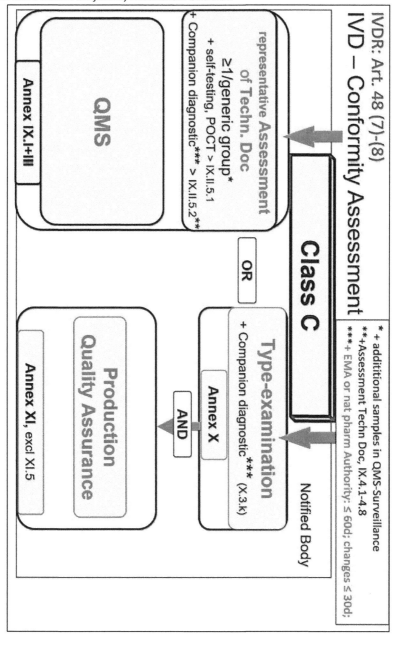

IVDR: Art. 48 (7)-(8)
IVD – Conformity Assessment

Class C

Annex IX.I+III

QMS

representative Assessment
of Techn. Doc
≥1/generic group*
+ self-testing, POCT > IX.II.5.1
+ Companion diagnostic*** > IX.II.5.2**

OR

Type-examination
+ Companion diagnostic *** (X.3.k)

Annex X

AND

Production
Quality Assurance

Annex XI, excl XI.5

Notified Body

* + additional samples in QMS-Surveillance
** +Assessment Techn Doc, IX.4.1-4.8
*** + EMA or nat pharm Authority: ≤ 60d; changes ≤ 30d;

13.6.3. IVD Conformity Assessment Class B:

(Fig. 43); According to IVDR: Art. 48 (9), Class B IVD manufacturers are subject to a conformity assessment of

> - **Annex IX, Chapt. I (QMS)[490] + III (administrative provisions)**
>
>   **AND**
>
> - **Annex IX, Chapt. II (Assessment of TD) acc to Annex IX.II.4.** for at least 1 representative example per device category[491]
>
>   **+ Annex IX.II.5.1 for IVD for self-testing and POCT**

---

[490] During surveillance audits the NB may draw further samples of TD per device category and assess the TD acc to Annex IX.II.4.; see also IVDR: Annex VII.4.5.2, 4th indent

[491] For sampling, see MDCG 2019-13: Guidance on sampling of devices for the assessment of the technical documentation

Fig. 43 IVDR: Class B Conformity Assessment Overview

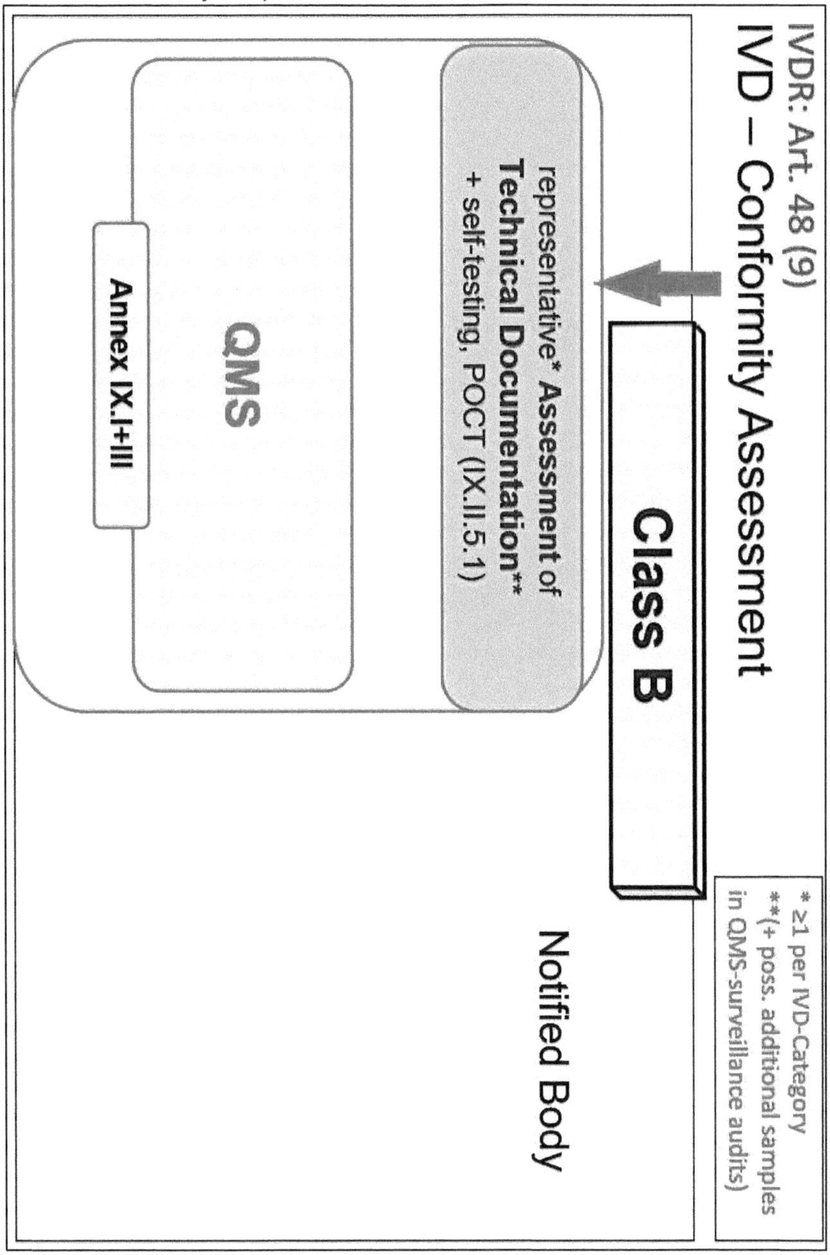

IVDR: Art. 48 (9)

IVD – Conformity Assessment

Class B

representative* Assessment of **Technical Documentation**** + self-testing, POCT (IX.II.5.1)

QMS

Annex IX.I+III

Notified Body

* ≥1 per IVD-Category
**(+ poss. additional samples in QMS-surveillance audits)

13.6.4. IVD Conformity Assessment Class A:

(Fig. 44); According to IVDR: Art. 48 (10), Class A IVD manufacturers are subject to conformity assessment according to

- **Annex II + III (draw up Technical Documentation)**

AND

- **EU-Declaration of Conformity** acc to Art. 17 and Annex IV by manufacturer[492]

AND

+ Annex IX (QMS) or Annex XI (Production Quality Assurance) for sterile Class A-IVDs[493]; these Annexes with notified body, limited to the aspects of establishing, securing and maintaining sterility

Conformity assessment for Class A non-sterile IVDs is performed by the manufacturer under his own responsibility, in particular on the basis of the preparation and updating of the Technical Documentation (TD) in accordance with Annexes II + III. In this case, the manufacturer is subject to random checks by competent authorities; in addition, the general manufacturer's obligations under Art. 10 of the IVDR must be fulfilled.

---

[492] These are anyhow part of the manufacturer's obligations under IVDR: Art. 10! Please be aware of the language requirements of the MSs where marketing is planned!
[493] Class A IVDs, placed on the market in sterile condition

Fig. 44 IVDR Class A Conformity Assessment Overview

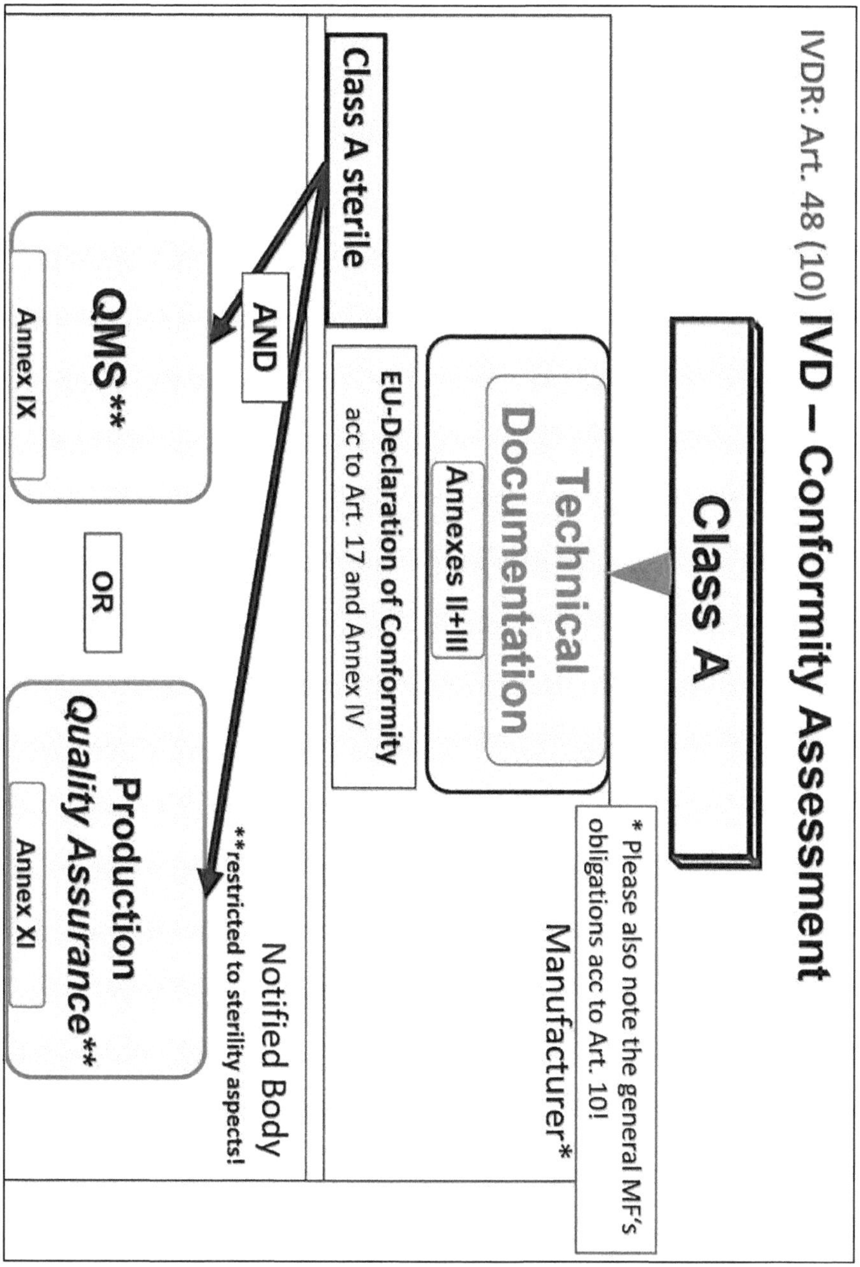

IVDR: Art. 48 (10) IVD – Conformity Assessment

Class A

Technical Documentation

Annexes II+III

EU-Declaration of Conformity
acc to Art. 17 and Annex IV

Class A sterile

AND

QMS*

Annex IX

OR

Production Quality Assurance*

Annex XI

Notified Body
**restricted to sterility aspects!

Manufacturer*

* Please also note the general MF's obligations acc to Art. 10!

For certain high-risk products, the assessment by the NB is supplemented by

13.7. Consultation Procedures

- for **Class D** by **European reference laboratories** (if available for the product type) to check for Performance claimed by the manufacturer and compliance with CS, if existing, within 60d, incl. lab testing. Additionally an **expert panel** has to be consulted (if no common specifications, CS, for this type of IVDs is available and where it is the first certification of such a product) within 60d; the EU reference laboratories will then also be consulted for certain planned changes (within 60d) to product and/or intended purpose, and for batch releases (within 30d). The scientific opinion of the EU reference laboratory is binding on the NB, i.e. the NB cannot issue a certificate if the scientific opinion is negative[494]!

- in the case of **companion diagnostics** by a competent authority for medicinal products (EMA or national)[495] within 60d, (possibly + a further 60d); or in the case of certain planned changes within 30d[496].

13.8. After Successful Conformity Assessment (Classes D - A)

If successful, the NB (for Class A sterile and higher Classes) issues the required (see also chapter I.2.4. in this book):

- **certificate(s)** (valid for a maximum of 5 years) and allow the manufacturer to affix its
- **NB's 4-digit identification number**, as a sign of successful "European Premarket Approval"

The manufacturer can then issue the

---

[494] See IVDR: Art. 48 (5+6) and Annex IX.II.4.9+11-13 and Annex X.3.(j). See also MDCG 2021-22: Clarification on "first certification for that type of device" and corresponding procedures to be followed by notified bodies, in context of the consultation of the expert panel referred to in Article 48(6) of Regulation (EU) 2017/746 and
MDCG 2021-4: Application of transitional provisions for certification of class D in vitro diagnostic medical devices according to Regulation (EU) 2017/746
[495] https://www.ema.europa.eu/en/human-regulatory/overview/medical-devices#companion-diagnostics-('in-vitro-diagnostics')-section
[496] See Art. 48 (7) 3rd subpara, and Annex IX.II.5.2 and Annex X.3.(k)

- **EU Declaration of Conformity** on that basis (for class A non-sterile on the manufacturer's own responsibility without the NB certificate!) in the required languages of the MS where the placing on the market is being planned and
- affix the **CE marking** (with the NB's 4 digit identification number (if a NB has been involved),
- and then start marketing[497]. Furthermore, if not already done before,
- the **registration obligations** and the **UDI obligations** according to the specific schedule (see chapter I.6 and IV of this book) must be fulfilled.

Conformity assessment is not a singular event; after successful certification it also includes regular, usually annual and also unannounced[498] **audits by the NB** and timely insight of the NB into current PMS and vigilance reports of the manufacturer. Furthermore, **planned changes** to the product, its intended purpose or the QMS are subject to evaluation by the notified body, which, depending on the scope and relevance of the **planned change**[499], may lead to a **supplement to the EU certificate** on the assessment of the TD or the QMS or the EU type examination, or to **a new conformity assessment** in accordance with Art. 48 of the MDR. A new consultation with consulted authorities may also be necessary.

Note: The general manufacturer's obligations with the life cycle processes (above all QMS, risk management, performance evaluation with PMPF, PMS and vigilance, registration obligations, traceability, communication with competent authorities and other stakeholders) remain in force in the further course (see Chapter 3.1. in this book)!

---

[497] Unless other legislations, which also apply to that product still have to be fulfilled
[498] At least once in 5 years
[499] See NBOG document NBOG BPG 2014-3: Guidance for manufacturers and Notified Bodies on reporting of Design Changes and Changes of the Quality System:
https://www.nbog.eu/nbog-documents/ :"It is recommended that manufacturers contact and discuss with their Notified Body about any questions related to the substantial or not substantial characteristic of the change in order to get
a common understanding."

In the case of **Class D IVDs**, an additional control mechanism (**Scrutiny procedure**) by Member States, COM and/or expert panel is also foreseen in accordance with Art. 50 (market surveillance immediately after certification).

Important: In contrast to IVD Directive 98/79/EC, the majority of IVDs are now subject to conformity assessment with notified bodies (NB) in the IVDR; therefore: search for and contract suitable notified body(s) for the new IVDR in good time! (Selection of NB, see chapter 13.4)

If you intend to use the prolonged transition periods under Amendment Regulation (EU) 2022/112 where your IVD did not need a NB under the IVDD and under the IVDR now would need one, **please assure, that you have issued your EU Declaration of Conformity (and other obligations of IVDD) before 26. May 2022!**

Chapter 14. Surveillance After the Start of Placing on the Market, Responsibilities

The new regulations also provide in their chapters VII - in accordance with the New Legal Framework for EU product legislation - for strengthened control instruments for the post-marketing phase of the MDs and IVDs, each with defined responsibilities (Tab. 23):

Tab. 23 MDR/IVDR: Surveillance after Placing on the Market/Putting into Service, Responsibilities

	Manufacturer	Competent Authority/COM
Post-Market Surveillance (PMS) (Chapt. VII.1)	X	
Vigilance (Chapt. VII.2)	X	X
Market Surveillance (Chapt. VII.3)		X

The respective manufacturer's obligations on PMS and Vigilance are monitored by their NB (if one is involved) esp. in the higher risk classes. Competent authorities will look at it in the course of market surveillance and esp. in case of (suspected) non-conformities. The European database EUDAMED will play a supporting role with its modules ("electronic systems") for PMS+Vigilance and Market Surveillance (see Fig. 12).

Chapter 15. Post-Market Surveillance (PMS), PMS System

15.1. Sources :

Legal texts:

- MDR/IVDR: Chapt. VII.1 and Annex III
- Also important for PMS:
  - UDI and Traceability: MDR/IVDR: Chapt. IV and Annex VI/C
  - PMCF[500]: MDR: Annex XIV.B
  - PMPF: IVDR: Annex XIII.B

Guidelines:

MDCG-Documents to UDI[501]:

MDCG-Documents zu PMCF:

MDCG 2020-8 Guidance on PMCF evaluation report template

MDCG 2020-7 Guidance on PMCF plan template

MEDDEV zu PMCF[502]:

MEDDEV 2.12/2 rev.2 Post market clinical follow-up studies (for MDR not up-to-date)

GHTF/IMDRF:

Guidelines for PMS are being developed at IMDRF-level, but are rather targeted to vigilance:

Medical Devices: Post-Market Surveillance: National Competent Authority Report Exchange, Criteria and Report Form (directed to vigilance system and deals with Global NCARs [National Competent Authority Reports], see chapter XVI in this book.

Standards:

ISO TR 20416: Medical devices – Post-market surveillance for manufacturers
(not yet harmonized to MDR/IVDR, but already now extremely useful for the build-up of a PMS-System, esp. for PMS-plans, with a lot of practical examples! Other parts of PMS under MDR/IVDR are currently lacking, like Periodic Safety Update Reports (PSURs) or PMS-reports.

---

[500] PMCF vs. PMPF are integral parts of the clinical evaluation of MDs vs. the performance evaluation of IVDs, but also of the PMS system (the part of the PMS that deals specifically with clinical data (MD) vs. performance data of IVDs).

[501] https://ec.europa.eu/health/md_sector/new_regulations/guidance_en

[502] https://ec.europa.eu/health/md_sector/current_directives_en

15.2. Survey of PMS-System

For each MD/IVD, manufacturers must plan, set up, document, apply, maintain and update a functional **PMS System** (Fig. 45) appropriate to the risk class and type of MD/IVD, based on a **PMS plan** (Annex III) for its life cycle under its mandatory QMS.

The main tasks of the PMS system for the respective MD/IVD are:

- To systematically collect and detect undesirable properties of the MD/IVD and its application, which had not (yet) been recognized until the completion of the (initial) conformity assessment, and to eliminate these immediately in order to rule out (further) undesirable risks for patients/users;

- Pro-actively and systematically collect, record and analyse **relevant data on the quality, safety and performance of the MD/IVD** (which parameters, indicators, thresholds? They have to be patient/user, product, application, production, servicing-relevant, comprehensive and measurable and be justified in the PMS-plan). These will have to be pro-actively collected throughout the life cycle of the MD/IVD and suitable to draw appropriate **conclusions** about possible CAPA[503]s, FSCA[504] s, improvement possibilities and on necessary updates to documents, including of the technical documentation, and

- To check the up-to-datedness of the previous assumptions and results of preclinical evaluation, clinical evaluation, risk management, the up-to-datedness of technical documentation, further compliance with the general safety and performance requirements, etc,

- identify, implement and monitor any need for improvements, corrections, CAPAs, FSCAs and inform the competent authorities and the NB thereof if indicated; and

- issue clear reports on the PMS data collected during the reporting period, their analysis, the results of the PMS system and the conclusions drawn and, if necessary, any corrective measures taken, in the form of

---

[503] CAPA: Corrective And Preventive Actions
[504] FSCA: Field Safety Corrective Action (like withdrawals and recalls)

(depending on the class of the MD/IVD) **PMS reports** or **Periodic Safety Update Reports (PSURs)**. (see Tab. 24)

15.3. The PMS Plan

The **PMS plan** is described in Annex III of the Regulations and would include (see also ISO TR 20416 for assistance):

- Clear description of MD/IVD in question, incl. variants, and intended purpose (should be in line with the Technical Documentation acc. to MDR/IVDR, Annex II.1, see chapter X. in this book;
- Clear objectives of PMS-system and PMS-plan;
- Responsibilities;
- PMS data collection:
    - A list of PMS information sources
    - methodology of PMS data collection;
    - protocols and templates for PMS data retrieval
- PMS data analysis (methodology and procedure part for active, systematic analysis of PMS information retrieved):
    - Key points of the analysis (parameters, benchmarks, thresholds, references etc. for the analysis with justification).
    - Planning of the data analysis (with comparisons, thresholds, time slots ... with justifications)
    - Results and reports on data analysis;
    - Method for drawing conclusions on possible improvements, CAPAs or FSCAs with implementation methodology;
    - Coordination with other processes (clinical evaluation, performance evaluation, RMS, TD, Vigilance, etc)
- References to the PMS reporting; formats, templates for PMS-reports, PSURs, trend reports, as applicable;
- a PMCF vs. PMPF plan (with a justification if this is not considered applicable; for PMCF please consider MDCG 2020-7: Guidance on PMCF plan template; MDCG 2020-8 Guidance on PMCF evaluation report template;

for PMPF: MDCG 2022-2: Guidance on general principles of clinical evidence for In Vitro Diagnostic medical devices (IVDs), chapter 7.

*A very valuable and practical help for setting up a PMS system under a QMS, under a PMS plan, has been developed within the framework of **ISO TR 20416 "Medical Devices – Post market surveillance for manufacturers"**. In addition to clear recommendations for setting up PMS plans for the manufacturer's medical devices and IVDs, there is comprehensive guidance on suitable data sources (Annex A, to be specified for the MD or IVD in question), on the appropriate methodology for evaluating PMS data (Annex B, also to be specified towards MD or IVD in question), and practical examples of PMS plans (Annex C, with indications on how to deal with specific product types of MDs and IVDs).*

Examples of possible PMS data sources
- Serious incidents (including info from PSURs) and FSCA information;
- Reports in data bases of competent authorities on serious incidents, FSCA, FSN concerning similar MDs/IVDs[505];
- Records of non-serious adverse events/reactions and any undesirable side-effects[506],
- Information from trend reporting,
- Publicly available information of similar MDs/IVDs;
- Relevant professional/specialist/technical literature, especially on current state of the art or changes thereto (like variants of SARS-Cov-2),
- Information, including feedbacks and complaints from patients, users, distributors, importers (with evaluation methodology);
- Relevant databases and/or registers, especially implant registers,
- Investigations of explants[507],

---

[505] See EUDAMED, when PMS+vigilance module is functional or FDA's MAUDE database

[506] In the analysis it will then be necessary to look whether there are indications for changes in kind, severity or probability of such events, in case of also with a reference to the denominator-function in the PSUR: Take into account that for the Periodic Safety Update Report (PSUR) according to the MDR: Art. 86 (1) (c) or IVDR: Art. 81 (1) (c) requires a denominator function of:

c) the total quantity of the product sold and an estimate of the number and

and other characteristics of the persons to whom the product in question is applied, and, where practicable, the frequency of use of the product.

[507] For the methodology, see e.g. the ISO/FDIS 12891 series of standards: Retrieval and analysis of surgical implants, also with the bibliography given there.

- Information from installation, maintenance, servicing, repairs, returns, reprocessing, from customer service, marketing,
- own hotlines with the corresponding feedbacks, reports retrieved,
- Public media, such as press, TV, radio, internet (e.g. official announcements, blogs, ...)
- Information from user or expert focus groups, patient or user blogs; interviews if necessary; Questionnaires; monitoring of user/patient groups and blogs;
- Information from training courses, simulation trainings, education etc
- feedback from the Customer Relationship Management (CRM),
- QA measures such as interlaboratory tests for IVDs, QA-testing, ring trials; acceptance tests or constancy tests in diagnostic imaging;
- Social media (assessment of the validity of the reported data ...)
- Internet research, for the indication areas
- Reports/questionnaires from user trainings and education;
- Market surveillance reports from the authorities with the associated results and recommendations
- Market observations of similar, comparable but also of novel medical devices/IVDs for the field of application;
- (Scientific) literature searches; if necessary, literature alerts set for updates on relevant questions in the initial literature searches;
- Reports from relevant conferences, trade fairs, training events, cluster meetings;
- Results of product approvals and tests; test reports; internal and external audits and inspections; also from sub-suppliers;
- PMCF studies/PMPF studies results and register evaluations.

15.4. PMS Data Analysis and Drawing Conclusions

These possible data sources are to be processed with a suitable **data analysis methodology**: In each case, it must be examined which sources, and how, are methodologically suitable as sources for **meaningful parameters, indicators or thresholds for the quality, safety and/or performance/effectiveness** of such medical devices/IVDs. How can these be traced in a proper methodology over defined and meaningful time slots (which have to be justified)? Other objectives and questions concern the analysis and evaluation of the current state of the art, and to what extent these parameters, indicators, thresholds, limit values etc may trace acceptability of the benefit/risk profile of the MD/IVD within PMCF/PMPF over a longer period of time. In addition, factors such as the quality and suitability of education, training, service and maintenance activities and, if applicable, of a Customer Relationship Management (CRM) is here at stake.

The necessary methods, protocols, instruments, questionnaires, literature searches, data mining etc. must be developed.

Suitable precautions for **product identification and traceability** are important (see chapter 4 in this book). Also important is a quantitative overview of products, attributed to e.g. batches, series, variants etc. but also the quantity of affected patients and users or number of applications (see denominator function for PSUR!), so that necessary searches or measures such as CAPAs or FSCAs can run smoothly and focused in the event of investigation of incidents or necessary measures.

Of course, the methodological tools can only be effective if, in addition to the necessary instruments,

- processes or protocols are in place,
- the staff concerned must be trained and
- assignment of responsibilities as well as competence among the staff concerned and
- the interfaces to other affected processes (e.g. clinical evaluation, performance assessment, risk management, research and development, regulatory, vigilance etc.)

are in place, and on that basis further necessary investigations, improvement processes, corrective and preventive actions, vigilance activities, like FSCA, may function smoothly and targeted.

15.5. PMS-Reporting

See Tab. 24 for low and higher risk MDs/IVDs. After actively and systematically collecting the relevant data and the appraisal and analysis of and drawing conclusions on these data following the PMS-plan, proper reporting is needed:

Tab. 24 MDR/IVDR: PMS-Reporting

PMS-Report[508]	Periodic Safety Update Report (PSUR)
MDR: Class I/IVDR: Class A+B	MDR: Class IIa-III/IVDR: Class C+D
• Summarize results and conclusions of analyses of PMS data • Rationale and description of any CA-PAs	• Summarize results and conclusions of analyses of PMS data • Rationale and description of any CA-PAs
	• Conclusions on the benefit/risk determination • Main findings of the PMCF/PMPF • Establish **denominator** functions: Volume of sales of MD/IVD; Estimate of size and characteristics of user population of device; Usage frequency of device
Frequency: updated when necessary; to Competent Authority on request	**Frequency: MD: IIb und III/IVD: C+D: at least annually** IIa: when necessary, but at least each 2nd year
	MDR: Implants + Class III/IVDR Class D: direct to EUDAMED: NB evaluates and uploads its assessment to EUDAMED: PSUR and its Assessment by NB are directly accessible to Competent Authorities (CAs) MDR: IIa + IIb (non-implants)/IVDR: Class C: PSUR always to NB, and to CAs on request

---

[508] See MDR: Art. 85/IVDR: 80; (PMS Report); PSUR: MDR: Art. 86/IVDR: 81

Fig. 45 PMS-System Overview

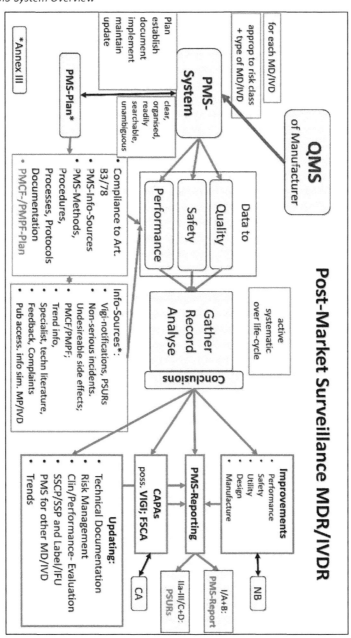

299

Chapter 16: The Vigilance System

16.1. Sources:

Legal basis:

Chapt. VII.2 of both Regulations

EU-Guidelines[509]:

MEDDEV 2.1.12 rev. 8 (still to be formally adapted to MDR/IVDR, but still functional also for the Regulations), subsequently for this chapter cited as MEDDEV;

• Additional Guidance Regarding the Vigilance System as outlined in MEDDEV 2.12-1 rev 8, subsequently for this chapter cited as Additional Guidance;

• New Forms at COM Homepage, esp.

  • **Manufacturer Incident Report (MIR);**
  • Form for Field Safety Corrective Action (FSCA);
  • Template for Field Safety Notice (FSN), incl. FSN Customer reply; FSN distributor/importer reply;

• Device Specific Vigilance Guidances (DSVG), currently for cardiac ablation, coronary stents, cardiac implantable electronic devices, breast implants, Insulin Infusion Pumps and Integrated meter systems.

IMDRF Guidance:

IMDRF terminologies for categorized Adverse Event Reporting (AER): terms, terminology, structure and codes, IMDRF/AE WG(PD1)/N43 FINAL:2019 (Edition 3): Guidance with the Terms und Codes for Annexes A-G, you will need for the Manufacturer Incident Report (MIR)

16.2. Survey of the Vigilance System

(see Fig. 46: Overview of EU vigilance system MDR/IVDR, Chapter VII.2.).

The vigilance system for the manufacturer is practically the tip of the "iceberg" of the Post Market Surveillance System (PMS) and focuses on the management of the most risky incidents for patients and, if applicable, users, or

---

[509] https://ec.europa.eu/health/sites/health/files/md_sector/docs/md_guidance_meddevs.pdf

After transfer into MDCG-Guidances these Guidelines will be found under: https://ec.europa.eu/health/md_sector/new_regulations/guidance_en

the most urgent corrective actions to prevent further similar incidents or hazardous situations.

The vigilance system is now also considered a **life cycle process** and an obligation of the manufacturer under Art. 10 , which he has to **operate under his QMS** and which is also closely linked to his **PMS system** (see chapter XV in this book) and to **traceability** (see chapter III in this book).

In Chapter VII.2, both Regulations have largely benefitted from the Guideline MEDDEV 2.12-1 rev 8, "Guidelines on a Medical Devices Vigilance System", which formally represents a detailed interpretation of the vigilance system of the previous 3 Medical Device Directives. Important parts and ideas of the rev 8 of the MEDDEV have now been incorporated into the formal rules of Section VII.2 of both regulations. Especially in the transition phase, one might be grateful to use the many practical notes, explanations, **checklists** and **forms** of the MEDDEV rev 8, even though formally one must always have a look at the text of the two Regulations.

1) At the core of the vigilance system is the **vigilance reporting**:

The following reporting obligations in the vigilance system result from the MDR/IVDR (the focus is on A) and B) below; see also left and middle column in Fig.46), for more detail see the surveys in Tab. 25 (short) and 26 (more detailed):

Tab. 25 MDR/IVDR: Short Survey of Reporting under Vigilance

A) The reporting of serious incidents
B) The reporting of field safety corrective actions (FSCA)
C) Other reporting obligations and variants, such as periodic summary reports, trend reports; user/patient reports;
D) Specific incidents, such as use errors and abnormal use.

Serious incidents[510] (via the **Manufacturer Incident Report – MIR**) and **field safety corrective actions (FSCA),** like e.eg. recalls or withdrawals, have to be reported via EUDAMED to the competent Authorities (CA) concerned. The new regulations now – like the MEDDEV - additionally contain <u>variants of vig-</u>

---

[510] See the definitions used within the vigilance system in chapter 16.3 of this book

ilance reports (Tab. 25 and 26), such as **periodic summary reports** (PSR; under defined conditions!), **trend reports** and provisions on **reports from health professionals, users and patients**.

2) The manufacturer, once aware of a serious incident, has an obligation to examine and critically analyse (root cause analysis) the serious incident and clarify a possible causal role of his MD/IVD in that incident, the possible risks and harms to be incurred by patients, users or ev. 3rd persons from possible reoccurrence of such incidents and to find the best remedial and preventative actions to be taken. In the course of his investigations, the manufacturer will, if necessary, have to issue follow-up reports to his initial MIR, and finally, with his conclusions and remedial actions a final MIR. Under remedial actions may also be **Field Safety Corrective Actions (FSCA**; e.g. withdrawals or recalls), which also have to be reported via EUDAMED to the Competent Authorities concerned. FSCAs will have to be accompanied by **Field Safety Notices (FSN)** to concerned distributors and users to enact all necessary safety measures.

The manufacturer will then have to monitor the success of his remedial actions.

The manufacturer will be assisted in his vigilance activities by his Person responsible for regulatory compliance (see MDR/IVDR: Art. 15 and MDCG 2019-7[511].

3) During his investigations and seek for remedial and preventative action, the manufacturer is under concurrent control by his Competent Authority (CA)[512]. The Competent Authority may perform its own investigations and remedial actions, if the manufacturer's actions are not deemed sufficient and timely enough. The Competent will usually have a critical look at all remedial and preventative actions planned by the manufacturer (esp. FSCAs) and indicate necessary changes before.

---

[511] MDCG 2019-7: Guidance on article 15 of the medical device regulation (MDR) and in vitro diagnostic device regulation (IVDR) on a 'person responsible for regulatory compliance' (PRRC)
[512] Sometimes several concerned CA will work together on that

4) Cooperation of MS: As serious incidents and FSCAs may concern several Member States (MS), the Competent Authorities of these concerned MS will usually work together in their control of the manufacturers vigilance activities. In the case of vigilance cases involving several Member States, the competent authorities can organise themselves under the leadership of a single coordinating national competent authority or as a vigilance task force, but without giving up their sovereignty and their own ability to act (see right column of Fig. 42). There may be a special data exchange between the authorities via EU-NCARs (EU-National Competent Authority Reports) or globally within the IMDRF via IMDRF NCARs (see right column Fig. 46).

Fig. 46 MDR/IVDR: Overview of Vigilance-System

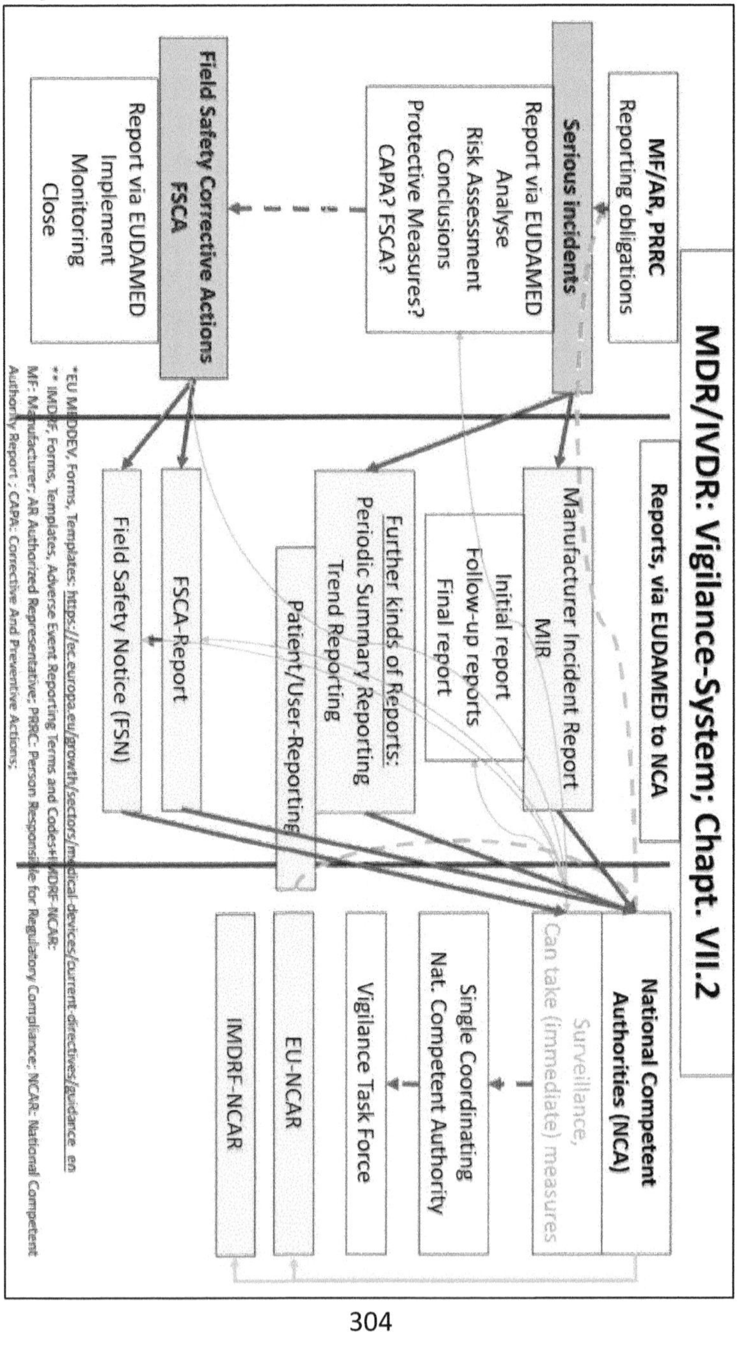

MDR/IVDR: Vigilance-System; Chapt. VII.2

MF/AR, PRRC
Reporting obligations

Serious incidents
Report via EUDAMED
Analyse
Risk Assessment
Conclusions
Protective Measures?
CAPA? FSCA?

Field Safety Corrective Actions
FSCA
Report via EUDAMED
Implement
Monitoring
Close

Reports, via EUDAMED to NCA

Manufacturer Incident Report
MIR
Initial report
Follow-up reports
Final report

Further kinds of Reports:
Periodic Summary Reporting
Trend Reporting

Patient/User-Reporting

FSCA-Report

Field Safety Notice (FSN)

National Competent Authorities (NCA)

Can take (immediate) measures
Surveillance,

Single Coordinating
Nat. Competent Authority

Vigilance Task Force

EU-NCAR

IMDRF-NCAR

* EU MEDDEV, Forms, Templates: https://ec.europa.eu/growth/sectors/medical-devices/current-directives/guidance_en
** IMDRF, Forms, Templates, Adverse Event Reporting Terms and Codes+IMDRF-NCAR:
MF: Manufacturer; AR Authorized Representative; PRRC: Person Responsible for Regulatory Compliance; NCAR: National Competent
Authority Report ; CAPA: Corrective And Preventive Actions;

16.3. The Manufacturer Incident Report - MIR

Serious incidents have to be reported by the **Manufacturer Incident**[513] **Report – MIR**. The New Manufacturer Incident Report (MIR), although still presented under the MEDDEV 2.12/1 rev.8, has already been adapted to MDR/IVDR on the COM homepage. See also the New Manufacturer Incident Report help text on the COM homepage[514].

> ## Please make yourself acquainted with the MIR[515] in advance!

This will be really important to avoid panic mode if a serious incident occurs! A lot of data (like data of the Competent Authorities within EU/EEA, important 3rd countries, like CH and UK, IMDRF; UDI; EMDN; risk classification; IMDRF-codes for adverse event reporting [see below]) should already be at hand to avoid painful seeking in an emergency situation! Please assure the necessary cooperation on that within your organisation, including the Person Responsible for Regulatory Compliance (PRRC), acc. To MDR/IVDR: Art. 15. Offline trainings on model cases corresponding to your product portfolio may be indicated ...

The structure of the MIR:

1. **Section 1: Administrative information**
    1.1. Corresponding Competent Authority
    1.2. Date, type and classification of incident report
    1.3. Submitter information
        1.3.1. Submitter of report

---

[513] Please note the difference in terminology: "Serious incident" under MDR/IVDR would correspond to "incident" under the Directives!

[514] https://ec.europa.eu/health/sites/health/files/md_sector/docs/md_guidance_meddevs.pdf

[515] The MIR reporting form distinguishes between the following types of reports for which this form can be used (please tick in each case!):
-Initial
-Follow up
-Combined initial and final
-Final (Reportable incident)
-Final (Non-reportable incident)

IMDRF Adverse Event Terms and Codes

For the understanding of the new MIR, the terminology of the IMDRF on Adverse Event Reporting "IMDRF terminologies for categorised Adverse Event Reporting (AER): terms, terminology, structure and codes[516] " is a prerequisite, for which manufacturers must now be prepared for.

The following annexes with coding in several levels are available:

The terminology for serious incidents (in IMDRF terminology: adverse events) outlined here consists of 3 main groups (see Fig. 47):

---

[516] IMDRF/AE WG/N43 FINAL:2021 Updated Annexes (Edition 5.0) http://www.imdrf.org/documents/documents.asp

- Observations at the level of the medical device, its components including accessories:
  - Annex A: Medical Device Problem Terms and Codes;
  - Annex G: Component Terms and Codes
- Investigation of possible causes of the event and causal relationships between the use of the medical device/IVD (whether or not there is a malfunction)
  - Annex B: Cause Investigation - Type of Investigation Terms and Codes
  - Annex C: Cause Investigation - Investigation Findings Terms and Codes
  - Annex D: Cause Investigation - Investigation Conclusion Terms and Codes
- Observations, typically adverse health effects, at the level of the affected persons, i.e. patients, users or other persons:
  - Annex E: Health Effects - Clinical Signs, Symptoms and Conditions Terms and codes
  - Annex F: Health Effects - Health Impact Terms and Codes

At the level of the individual annexes, there are up to 3 hierarchical levels of codes; try to code as deeply as possible and include this in the appropriate positions in the MIR at the appropriate positions. (Overview IMDRF AER Terms and Codes, see Fig. 47 IMDRF Adverse Events Terms and Codes)

Fig. 47 IMDRF Adverse Event Terms and Codes

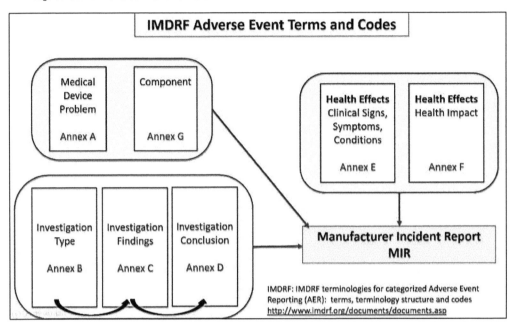

It is particularly important for manufacturers and the departments and persons responsible for vigilance (also PRRC!) to be aware of the data requirements and procedures (English language skills!!) for this MIR form and with the corresponding IMDRF codes in good time, also in offline exercises, in advance. You should be aware which data for such reports on serious incidents must be kept available at all times. Test this offline with data from freely available data on such incidents (e.g. from publicly available FSNs, see linklist)

Please make yourself familiar with the IMDRF-codes in advance!

For reporting obligations in detail, see chapter 16.4. and Tab. 26 below:

Kind of Report	Explanation; Specification, when to choose?	Sources in MDR/IVDR and MEDDEV
Individual reporting: Serious Incident	any serious incident, i.e. an incident that directly or indirectly led, might have led or might lead to any of the following: (a) the death of a patient, user or other person, (b) the temporary or permanent serious deterioration of a patient's, user's or other person's state of health[517],	Art. 87/82 (1)a); MEDDEV Form MIR Annex 3;

---

[517] See clarification in MEDDEV 2.12-1 rev 8, 5.1.1.:

A **serious deterioration in state of health** can include (non-exhaustive list):

a) life-threatening illness,

b) permanent impairment of a body function or permanent damage to a body structure,

c) a condition necessitating medical or surgical intervention to prevent a) or b).

Examples:

- clinically relevant increase in the duration of a surgical procedure,

- a condition that requires hospitalization or significant prolongation of existing hospitalization.

d) any **indirect harm** (see definition under section 4.11 of MEDDEV; see also below) as a consequence of an incorrect diagnostic or IVD test result or as a consequence of the use of an IVF/ART device when used within MANUFACTURER's instructions for use (use errors reportable under section 5.1.5.1 of the MEDDEV must also be considered).

e) fetal distress, fetal death or any congenital abnormality or birth defects.

NOTE :

Not all (*serious – inclusion by author*) INCIDENTs lead to death or serious deterioration in health. The non-occurrence of such a result might have been due to other fortunate circumstances or to the intervention of healthcare personnel. It is sufficient that:

a (serious) INCIDENT associated with a device happened, and

the (serious) INCIDENT was such that, if it occurred again, it might lead to death or serious deterioration in health.

For IVDs and IVF/ART the concept of indirect harm is particularly important: see MEDDEV: 4.11 **INDIRECT HARM:**

In the majority of cases, diagnostic devices IVDs and IVF/ART medical devices will, due to their intended use, not directly lead to physical injury or damage to health of people (HARM

	(c) a serious public health threat;	
Field safety corrective action – FSCA	means corrective action taken by a manufacturer for technical or medical reasons to prevent or reduce the risk of a serious incident in relation to a device made available on the market[518];	Art. 87/82 (1)b); MEDDEV 5.4.4; Form Annex 4; FSN template An- nex 5;
Periodic Summary Re- ports – PSR	For similar serious incidents that occur with the same device or device type and ■ for which the root cause has been identified or ■ a field safety corrective action im- plemented or ■ where the incidents are common and well documented,	Art. 87/82 (9); Art.92(8)/Art .87(8) MEDDEV 5.1.2; Form Annex 6;

– see section 4.8 of MEDDEV). These devices are more likely to lead to indirect harm rather than to direct harm. HARM may occur as a consequence of the medical decision, action taken/not taken on the basis of information or result(s) provided by the device or as a conse- quence of the treatment of cells (e.g. gametes and embryos in the case of IVF/ART devices) or organs outside of the human body that will later be transferred to a patient.

Examples of indirect harm include
- misdiagnosis,
- delayed diagnosis,
- delayed treatment,
- inappropriate treatment,
- absence of treatment
- transfusion of inappropriate materials.

Indirect harm may be caused by
- imprecise results
- inadequate quality controls
- inadequate calibration
- false positive or
- false negative results.

[518] including any field safety corrective action undertaken in a third country in relation to a device which is also legally made available on the Union market, if the reason for the field safety corrective action is not limited to the device made available in the third country.

	the manufacturer may provide periodic summary reports instead of individual serious incident reports, on condition that the coordinating competent authority referred to in Art. 89(9)/84(9), in consultation with the competent authorities referred to in point (a) of Art. 92(8)/87(8), has agreed with the manufacturer on the format, content and frequency of the periodic summary reporting.	
Trend reporting	any statistically significant increase in the frequency or severity of incidents that are not serious incidents or that are expected undesirable side-effects that could have a significant impact on the benefit-risk analysis and which have led or may lead to risks to the health or safety of patients, users or other persons that are unacceptable when weighed against the intended benefits[519].	Art. 88/83; MED-DEV4.18;5.1. 4; Ann 1; Form: Annex 7;
Reports by healthcare professionals, users or patients	Reports on suspected serious incidents go to Competent Authority (CA), which transmits it without delay to MF. MF shall report it as individual serious incident report via EUDAMED to CA or (if not considered a serious incident) use it in his PMS. CA may however demand serious incident report and possibly FSCA, if indicated.	Art. 87/82 (10), (11);

[519]The significant increase shall be established in comparison to the foreseeable frequency or severity of such incidents in respect of the device, or category or group of devices in question during a specific period as specified in the technical documentation and product information.

16.4. The reporting obligations in the vigilance system in detail[520]

16.4.1 Reporting of serious incidents

16.4.1.1 The obligation to report

Any serious incident related to medical devices/IVDs, made available on the Union market shall be reported through the electronic system.

There is a specific reporting form for this purpose (Manufacturer Incident Report, MIR).

Expected side-effects (IVDR: and expected erroneous results) are excluded from such reports, if they are

- clearly documented in the product information and quantified in the technical documentation, and are

- subject to the reporting of trends in accordance with Art. 88/83 of the Regulations.

16.4.1.2 Definitions

The following definitions in the regulations or the MEDDEV are important[521]:

'incident' means any malfunction or deterioration in the characteristics or performance of a device made available on the market, including use-error due to ergonomic features, as well as any inadequacy in the information supplied by the manufacturer and any undesirable side-effect;

'serious incident' means any incident that directly or indirectly led, might have led or might lead to any of the following:

(a) the death of a patient, user or other person,

(b) the temporary or permanent serious deterioration of a patient's, user's or other person's state of health,

(c) a serious public health threat;

---

[520] See also Tab. 26

[521] Note: The terminology of the MDR/IVDR differs from that of the MEDDEV in this respect: "incident" of the MDR/IVDR would correspond to the "event" of the MEDDEV, whereas "serious incident" of the MDR/IVDR corresponds to the "incident" of the MEDDEV.

'serious public health threat' means an event which could result in imminent risk of death, serious deterioration in a person's state of health, or serious illness, that may require prompt remedial action, and that may cause significant morbidity or mortality in humans, or that is unusual or unexpected for the given place and time;

"serious deterioration of health" MEDDEV (Chap. 5.1.1 C) explains:

[= non-exhaustive list of situations covered]:

a) Life-threatening illness,

b) permanent impairment of a body function or permanent damage to a body structure,

(c) a condition requiring medical or surgical intervention in order to prevent a) or b);

Examples:

clinically relevant prolongation of the duration of a surgical procedure,

a condition requiring hospitalisation or significant prolongation of an existing hospital stay

(d) any indirect harm resulting from an incorrect diagnostic result of an MD or IVD procedure or as a consequence of the use of an MD for IVF/ART when used within the scope of the manufacturer's instructions for use (which also includes application errors as defined in chap. 5.1.5.1. of the MEDDEV); in the majority of cases, diagnostic MDs, IVDs or MDs for IVF/ART, according to their intended purpose, will not directly cause physical injury or damage to the human health. Their hazard potential will mostly be of an indirect nature, whether as a consequence of faulty medical decisions, treatments or non-treatments based on faulty diagnoses, or as a consequence of the treatment of cells/tissues (e.g. gametes or embryos in the case of IVF/ART-MP) or organs outside the human body, which are then transferred to a patient.

Examples of indirect harm may include: misdiagnosis, delayed diagnosis, delayed treatment, inadequate choice of treatment, omission of treatment, transfusion of inappropriate material;

Indirect harm can be caused by, for example:

Inaccurate results, inadequate quality control or calibration, false positive or false negative results.

e) Foetal distress, foetal death or any congenital abnormality(ies) or birth defect(s).

16.4.1.3. Check whether there is the obligation to report serious incidents

MEDDEV 2.1.12 rev. 8 proposes the following **3 basic reporting criteria**, including explanations and examples, about the examination of any obligation to report serious incidents:

A) There is an incident[522]:
This can be among other things:
a) a malfunction or deterioration of the characteristics or performance of the MD/IVD: this should be understood as misconduct of an MD/IVD to perform the service in accordance with the intended purpose if it is used according to the manufacturer's instructions. It may also concern situations where the MD/IVD is subjected to tests, e.g. in quality control, or the information provided with the MD/IVD is examined or scientific information indicates a factor that could lead or has led to an incident.
b) Unforeseen adverse reactions or unforeseen side effects;
c) interactions with other substances or products;
d) Degradation or destruction of the MD/IVD (e.g. fire, e.g. batteries exploding);
e) Inappropriate therapy;
f) inaccuracies in labelling, instructions for use or advertising material (including omissions or deficits, unless this is information which should be generally known to the intended user);
g) For IVDs, all false positive or false negative test results should be considered incidents, and as serious incidents where there is a risk that an erroneous result may either:

---

[522] Please note a **difference in terminology between the Regulations and the MEDDEV**: The Regulations use: incident – serious incident, whereas the same in the MEDDEV is: event – incident! Here we follow the terminology of the Regulations.

(1) lead to a decision in patient management that leads to an immediate life-threatening situation of the tested person, or

(2) causes death or severe disability in the tested individual or fetus or to the individual's offspring;

h) Similarly, for IVDs, any false positive or negative results outside the performance claimed by the manufacturer should be considered as incidents.

B) The **MD/IVD of the manufacturer is suspected to have contributed causally to the incident or a causal relationship seems to be reasonably possible**[523]:

Here the manufacturer has to assess the possible link between the device and the incident; it should consider also evidence-based opinions of healthcare professionals, the results of his own investigations and assessments of the incident, the evidence from previous, similar incidents or other related findings. In case of doubt at least a preliminary notification is indicated, if also C) applies.

C) The incident has led or could have led to one of these consequences (= serious!):

- Death of a patient, user or other person;
- serious deterioration of the state of health of a patient, user or another person[524];
- Serious threat to public health.

16.4.1.4. Time limits for reporting serious incidents[525]

As a matter of principle, notification must be made immediately after the manufacturer has established a reasonably possible causal link between the incident and his product.

---

[523] Wording follows here MDR: Art. 87.3 and IVDR: Art. 82.3; the MEDDEV says:
B) The MF's device is suspected to be a contributory cause of the incident
[524] See MEDDEV 2.12-1 rev 8, 5.1.1.; see also Tab. 26, above
[525] MDR: Art. 87 (2)-(7); IVDR: Art. 82 (2)-(7)

However, the maximum time periods allowed by the MDR/IVDR after the manufacturer has become aware of the incident depend on the severity of the serious incident:

- In the event of a <u>serious public health threat</u>, immediately, but no later than **2 days** after the knowledge of the danger;
- In the event of <u>death</u> or an <u>unforeseen serious deterioration in the state of health</u> of a person, immediately, at the latest, however, **10 days** after becoming aware of the occurrence.
- Otherwise, no later than **15 days** after becoming aware of the incident[526];

In order to ensure prompt notification, the manufacturer may initially make a preliminary report, which he shall then follow up with a full report.

If the manufacturer is in doubt (uncertain) as to whether a report must be made, he should in any event rather report within the above-mentioned deadlines.

If a serious incident occurs in connection with the use of several medical devices/IVDs from different manufacturers, each of these manufacturers should submit a report.

The reporting of serious incidents does not per se imply for the manufacturer automatically assume liability for the incident and its consequences, the causes of which must first be investigated. The manufacturer will often add a disclaimer of liability to the (initial) report.

16.4.1.5. Final Report of the Manufacturer[527]

A final report with reference to the initial and any subsequent Follow-up vigilance reports shall be provided by the manufacturer via the EUDAMED electronic system. This report presents the results of the investigations, the conclusions drawn and the corrective and preventive actions to be taken (CAPA, FSCA, if indicated).

---

[526] Please note the difference to the MEDDEV, which had a time limit of 30 days here
[527] MDR: Art. 89 (5); IVDR: Art. 84 (5)

The form in Annex 3 of the MEDDEV may also be used until new electronic forms are available acc. to the regulations.

16.4.2. Field Safety Corrective Action (FSCA)

16.4.2.1. Reporting Obligation for FSCA

There is a reporting obligation for FSCA for medical devices/IVDs made available on the Union market.

This also includes FSCAs in third countries concerning medical devices/IVDs that are also made available on the Union market, unless the reason for such FSCA is exclusively local to the third country for the medical devices/IVDs made available there.

The manufacturer must not only report serious incidents but also investigate and, if necessary, take appropriate corrective measures. These corrective measures, such as FSCA, have to be taken to eliminate or reduce as far as possible the risk of death and serious harm to health, as well as serious risks to public health. FSCAs can help to prevent direct or indirect (e.g. due to erroneous results of diagnostic medical devices or IVDs) and must be reported by the manufacturer.

FSCAs must be reported in advance (before the safety measure is taken in the field) without undue delay, except in cases of urgency, where the manufacturer must take the FSCA immediately. In this case, he shall report as soon as possible.

16.4.2.2. Definitions of MDR/IVDR for FSCA[528]

'**corrective action**' means action taken to eliminate the cause of a potential or actual non-conformity or other undesirable situation;

'**field safety corrective action**' means corrective action taken by a manufacturer for technical or medical reasons to prevent or reduce the risk of a serious incident in relation to a device made available on the market;

'**field safety notice**' means a communication sent by a manufacturer to users or customers in relation to a field safety corrective action;

---

[528] MDR: Art. 2 (62)-(63), (67)-(69); IVDR: Art.2 (65)-(66), (70)-(72)

'**recall**' means any measure aimed at achieving the return of a device that has already been made available to the end user;

'**withdrawal**' means any measure aimed at preventing a device in the supply chain from being further made available on the market;

16.4.2.3. Examples of FSCA

(see MEDDEV, chapt. 4.6.) FSCA can include (see Additional Guidance, sec. 2.1, Notes 1-6):

- Recall;
- Withdrawal;
- MP/IVD Modification[529];
- Exchange of medical device/IVD;
- Destruction of medical device/IVD;
- Retrofitting at the instigation of the manufacturer;
- instructions/recommendations of the manufacturer regarding the use of the MP/IVD or the follow-up of patients (e.g. implant carriers, incorrect test results from IVD etc), users or third parties;[530]

---

[529] A modification may include:

Changes to labelling or instructions for use;

software upgrades as a result of the discovery of bugs in the software version already in the field; according to Note 2 of the Additional Guidance, this may also include the following modifications:

- advice relating to a change in the way the device is used, e.g. MANUFACTURER advises revised quality control procedure such as use of third party controls or more frequent calibration or modification of control values for the device,
- changes to storage conditions for sample to be used with an IVD,
- advice issued to USERs relating to a change in the stated shelf life of an IVF/ART device, e.g. IVF/ART MANUFACTURER informs USERs of an error on the labelling of his device which indicates a shelf life longer than the validated shelf life for the product;
- software upgrades following the identification of a fault in the software version already in the field (This should be reported regardless of whether the software update is being implemented by customers, field service engineers or by remote access.)

[530] Acc. to Note 4 of the Additional Guidance this could include:

- A serious defect discovered in the course of the manufacturer's QA activities or discovered during an inspection of a manufacturing site, which may have FSCA-required consequences and which may also affect medical devices already on the market[531].

Important: It is both the nature of the action taken, and the reason giving rise to the need for the action which defines whether an action is a FSCA.

FSCAs are notified to the competent authorities under the MDR/IVDR via EU-DAMED.
Until EUDAMED is operational, a notification form for FSCAs is available under the MEDDEV, Annex 4, a notification form for FSCAs is available for the Competent Authorities (CAs) concerned, including the CA where the manufacturer or his Authorised representative is established:

16.4.2.4. Minimum Content of an FSCA (Forms)
The FSCA notification according to Annex 4 of the MEDDEV should address all relevant aspects and include documents required by the competent authorities concerned to monitor the FSCA (according to MEDDEV, Chap. 5.4.4.1[532]); see also the Additional Guidance and the template for an FSCA notification of the COM.

Advice given by the MANUFACTURER may include modification to the clinical management of patients/samples to address a risk of death or serious deterioration in state of health related specifically to the characteristics of the medical device.
For example:
- for implantable devices it is often clinically unjustifiable to explant the device:
Corrective action taking the form of special patient follow-up, irrespective of whether any affected un-implanted devices remain available for return, constitutes FSCA.
- for diagnostic devices (e.g. IVD, imaging equipment or devices), corrective action
taking the form of the recall of patients or patient samples for retesting or the review of previous results constitutes FSCA
[531] See Note 2 of the Additional Guidance, chap. 2.1.; acc to Note 2 this may also concern certain Software Anomalies (e.g. incorrect correlation between
patient sample and the obtained result), or invalid controls, invalid calibrations or reagent failures (e.g. contamination, transcription errors and reduced stability).
[532] Under MDR/IVDR to supplemented by UDI and SRN

Minimum contents of an FSCA if template of the COM is not used:

- Relevant parts of the risk analysis;
- Background information and justification for the FSCA;
- Description and justification of the measure (corrective/preventive);
- Indication of the measures to be taken by the supplier and the user
- Precise identification of the medical devices/IVDs concerned, if available incl. UDI;
- If applicable, explanation of why other batches, serial numbers, etc. are not affected;
- Identification of the manufacturer/authorised representative, in case of availability incl. Single Registration Number, SRN;
- Copy of the Field Safety Notice, FSN

16.4.2.5. Field Safety Notice (FSN)

The manufacturer shall communicate an FSCA to users and suppliers via Field Safety Notices (FSN).

The MEDDEV provides a **template for a Field Safety Notice (FSN)** in Annex 5. and a **customer reply form** and an **importer/distributor reply form** are now available on the COM homepage.[533]

An FSN should, as far as possible, be designed in the same way for all EEA Member States concerned, unless a local situation requires otherwise; in any case, observe the nationally required language regime!

The distribution of the FSN should reflect the distribution and the user groups involved and should, if possible, be checked with confirmations of receipt.

(see customer reply form and distributor reply form, mentioned above)

16.4.2.6. Minimum Content of a Field safety Notice (FSN)

(MDR/IVDR; MEDDEV, Chap. 5.4.4.2 and Annex 5; Additional Guidance; Template of the COM):

Minimum content of an FSN if template is not used

---

[533] https://ec.europa.eu/docsroom/documents/32301/attachments/2/translations/en/renditions/pdf

- Clear title: Urgent Field Safety Notice, with commercial name and type of product;
- Identification of FSCA; and type of FSCA (e.g. recall etc);
- Specific details on the identification of affected medical devices/IVDs, type and model, batches, serial numbers etc., incl. UDI if available;
- Identification of the manufacturer with name and contact details, incl. SRN, if applicable other economic operators involved;
- Explanation of reasons for FSCA, incl. description of medical device/IVD defects or malfunctions and clarification of possible hazards to patients, users or third parties through further use, including, if applicable risks to patients arising from previous use of the medical devices/IVDs involved;
- Advice to users on measures to be taken, including, if necessary,
    - Identification and quarantine of the medical devices/IVDs;
    - Methods for safeguarding, disposal or modification;
    - Recommended follow-up for patients, especially also for implants and IVDS;
    - Indication that they or their health care institutions/professionals must be informed;
    - Timeline for action;
- Note that FSN is to be passed on to those who have been supplied with the medical device/IVD, who have the medical device/IVD;
- Note that these should be made known to the manufacturer for direct information on the FSCA and performance control!
- Confirmation that the competent authorities have been informed and involved about FSCA; and
- Contact details for the manufacturer's contact person/authorised representative for this FSCA.

All attempts to downplay risks or to use the FSCA for advertising purposes are to be refrained from!

16.4.3. Further Variants of Vigilance Reports

16.4.3.1. Periodic Summary Reports (PSR)

The above-mentioned vigilance reports of serious incidents are usually individual reports. Under certain conditions, **periodic summary reports (PSR)**[534] are also possible, namely with regard to similar serious incidents involving the same medical device/IVD or the same type of product,

- the cause of which has already been established, or
- for which an FSCA has already been made, or
- which occur frequently and are well documented (common and well documented).

if the manufacturer has agreed with the coordinating competent authority and the other authorities concerned on the **form, content and frequency of the periodic reports**.[535]

A form for periodic reports can be found in Annex 6 of the MEDDEV.2.12-1 rev 8.

With regard to certain product groups (currently these are Cardiac ablation; coronary stents; Cardiac implantable electronic devices (CIED), breast implants, Insulin Infusion Pumps and Integrated meter systems) there are Device Specific Vigilance Guidances (DSVG) with specific recommendations for possible periodic summary reporting prepared (see chapter 16.7. in this book). Make sure however with your competent authority whether this is acceptable.

16.4.3.2. Trend Reports

Manufacturers must also report via the EUDAMED electronic system:
Any statistically significant increase in the frequency or severity of

- of non-serious events or
- expected adverse reactions,

---

[534] MDR: Art. 86 (9) and IVDR: Art. 81 (9)
[535] Maybe only 1 Competent Authority is concerned, then the agreement on PSR is to be taken with that one

that could have a significant impact on the risk-benefit analysis according to Annex I, and which could result in risks to the health or safety of patients, users or other persons. [IVDR: or a significant increase in expected erroneous results compared to the declared performance of the IVD in accordance with IVDR: Annex I, Section 9.1(a) and (b) and as indicated in the technical documentation and product information which are unacceptable in view of the intended benefits. To this end, the manufacturer shall specify (and justify) the methodology for the detection of such increases and the choice of time periods in the PMS plan.

The significance of the increase shall be determined by comparison with the frequency or severity of such events in relation to the medical device/IVD concerned or the category or group of such devices, which are expected to occur within a given period of time and which is indicated in the technical documentation and product information.

The competent authorities may carry out their own investigations and assessments of trend reports and require the manufacturer to take appropriate measures in accordance with the with the Regulations to ensure the protection of public health and patient safety.

The COM, the other competent authorities and
the NB must be informed.

With regard to certain product groups (currently these are Cardiac ablation; coronary stents; Cardiac implantable electronic devices (CIED), breast implants and Insulin Infusion Pumps and integrated meter systems) there are Device Specific Vigilance Guidances (DSVG) with specific recommendations for periodic summary reporting and trend reporting. However, check with your competent authority whether this is acceptable.

16.4.3.3. Reports from health professionals, users and patients:
Member States are required to make these groups of people aware of the importance of their reporting of suspected serious incidents and to encourage them to do so.

Such reports should be collected centrally by the relevant competent authorities of the Member States and forwarded to the manufacturer without delay.

The manufacturer examines the reports and uses these reports in accordance with his obligation to notify, i.e. he makes an "official" report of a serious incident via the electronic system.

If the manufacturer is of the opinion that it is not a reportable incident, but a matter for the PMS, he shall inform the competent authority thereof with reasons. The competent authority may concur with the manufacturer's opinion or, if it does not agree with the manufacturer's conclusion, require the manufacturer to submit a report and to take follow-up action in the form of further analysis, risk assessment and FSCA as appropriate.

16.4.3.4. Special Occurrences: (Use Errors and Abnormal Use)

Such events, which become known to the manufacturer, must also be carefully recorded and evaluated. In these cases, the manufacturer must in any case check whether labelling and instructions for use are adequate. In addition, processes in risk management, PMS, usability, design validation, CAPA processes and user training. The results should be made available to the competent authorities and NB on request.

Use Errors to be reported:

Use Errors relating to medical devices/IVDs that result in death, serious serious deterioration in health or a serious risk to public health must be reported in any case.

Use Errors are also reportable to the competent authority ("supra-threshold"), if the manufacturer notices

- a significant change in the trend (esp. increase in frequency) or a significant change in the pattern of use errors,

that could potentially lead to such serious consequences, or if he

- initiates an FSCA in this context to prevent such severe consequences.

prevent such serious consequences.

Use errors that are not usually reportable:

Use errors involving medical devices/IVDs that have not led to the above serious consequences do not have to be reported, but are very much the subject of sincere considerations in the QMS, risk management and PMS.

Related decisions not to report must be justified and documented.

Furthermore, such occurrence captured in Trend reporting (see above) can become "overthreshold" in terms of reporting.

Considerations on abnormal use:

According to the MEDDEV, such events are not reportable in the vigilance system. Nevertheless, a "soul-searching" of the manufacturer is indicated, whether he has not contributed perhaps unintentionally to such events by certain elements (e.g. labelling, instructions for use, inadequate user training, misleading advertising, design errors, etc.),

If necessary, other competent authorities outside of the medical device/IVD sector, relevant health care institutions, bodies that carry out supervision, should be made aware of serious misconduct.

This is not least also in the interest of the manufacturer, who can thus avoid an unjustified bad reputation for its medical devices/IVDs in the public eye.

16.5. Forms, Contact data for vigilance

In the MEDDEV and at the COM-homepage you may find electronic report forms, templates and contact data for the vigilance system.

16.5.1. Forms, Templates and help texts at the COM-homepage[536]

• Report Form: Manufacturer's Incident Report (MIR),
now for MDR/IVDR: New MIR under the MEDDEVs at COM homepage!
• see also new MIR help text, very useful for filling out MIR
• Report Form: Manufacturer's Field Safety Corrective Action Report
• Template for a Field Safety Notice
• FSN customer reply
• FSN distributor/importer reply
• FSN Q&A
• Report Form: Manufacturer's Periodic Summary Report (PSR)
• Report Form: Manufacturer's Trend Report
• National Competent Authority Report (NCAR): This form will be used by the National Competent Authorities participating in the EU- and IMDRF[537] exchange program.

16.5.2. Contact details of the competent authorities for vigilance in the EEA

(CH, TK and UK to be checked separately, still 3rd country status?):

---

[536] Keep an eye on any new forms and templates that may be created in the course of adapting the vigilance guideline to the new regulations! It is to be expected
that in the new EUDAMED, PMS and Vigilance module, the forms can be filled in directly online. At present, these are listed under old Guidance: https://ec.europa.eu/health/sites/health/files/md_sector/docs/md_guidance_meddevs.pdf
In the course of further formal adaptation to MDR/IVDR, they could
they could be found under new Guidance as MDCG Documents: https://ec.europa.eu/growth/sectors/medical-devices/new-regulations/guidance_en
[537] http://www.imdrf.org/documents/documents.asp

See EU-COM homepage: Vigilance contact points: https://ec.europa.eu/health/sites/health/files/md_sector/docs/md_vigilance_contact_points.pdf

When the EUDAMED of the MDR/IVDR (module PMS and Vigilance) is operational, these notifications are submitted electronically and are automatically sent to the competent authorities concerned.

16.6. Exchange of information by the competent authorities

(National Competent Authorities, NCA).
The national competent authorities of the EU work closely together in the context of managing vigilance agendas (see right column in Fig. 46 Overview EU vigilance system, see also MDR/IVDR and Additional Guidance, section 8). This includes, under certain conditions, EU authorities' own reports to each other, so-called EU NCARs.

16.6.1 EU NCARs (EU National Competent Authority Reports).

These are usually made via EUDAMED, if functional, otherwise via the existing reporting channels in the current system.
EU NCARs are usually sent in the following situations:
- An FSCA is carried out by the MANUFACTURER;
- When a national competent authority requests the MANUFACTURER to perform an FSCA or requests to make changes to an FSCA that the MANUFACTURER is has already initiated;
- If there is a serious risk to the safety of patients or other USERS, but no corrective action has yet been taken, although it is being considered;
- When the MANUFACTURER fails to submit a final report in a timely manner.

For more detailed considerations on these EU NCARs, see the Additional Guidance, Sect. 8.

16.6.2. Single Coordinating Competent Authority and Vigilance Task Forces

If, due to the complexity or brisance of a vigilance case, several member states are involved in a vigilance operation, there is the possibility to set up a Single Coordinating Competent Authority.

Their selection, tasks and modalities of implementation can be found in MDR: Art. 89 (9)-(11) or IVDR: Art. Art. 84 (9)-(11) and in the Additional Guidance, Section 7.

The coordinating competent authority shall, through the electronic system referred to in Article 92 (MDR)/Art. 87 (IVDR), inform the manufacturer, the other competent authorities and the Commission that it has assumed the role of coordinating authority.

In very difficult and complex vigilance situations, the member states may also set up a **vigilance task force**. The composition, tasks and modalities of implementation are described in the Additional Guidance, section 7.2.

16.6.3. IMDRF NCAR Exchange

If an EU Member State considers that a vigilance report should be shared with a wider international regulatory community within the IMDRF, under certain conditions, this can be done in the framework of IMDRF NCARs. Modalities and forms can be found in IMDRF Document:

IMDRF/NCAR WG/N14 FINAL:2017 (Edition 2) "Medical Devices: Post-Market Surveillance: National Competent Authority Report; Exchange Criteria and Report Form[538]".

EU Member States wishing to participate in the IMDRF NCAR must qualify for it. (e.g. training; mutual confidentiality agreements). See also the Additional Guidance, section 9.

---

[538] http://www.imdrf.org/docs/ghtf/final/sg2/technical-docs/ghtf-sg2-n79r11-medical-devices-post-market-surveillance-090217.pdf#search=%22National%20Competent%20Authority%20Report;%20Exchange%20Criteria%20and%20Report%20Form%22

16.7. Product (group)-specific guidelines on vigilance

(Device Specific Vigilance Guidance; DSVG[539])

Please note that for specific kinds of (usually high risk) products a new format of **Device Specific Vigilance Guidance** (DSVG) is being made available. A template, an introductory guidance on DSVG and DSVGs on 5 high risk device groups are available. These will e.g. give clear hints, when individual serious incident reporting, summary reports and trend reporting are indicated. If in doubt on that, agreement should be reached thereon with the competent authority on the procedure to be chosen.

EU device specific vigilance guidance available:

DSVG Template

DSVG 00 Introduction to device specific vigilance guidance

DSVG 01 Cardiac ablation vigilance reporting guidance

DSVG 02 Coronary stents vigilance reporting guidance

DSVG 03 Cardiac implantable electronic devices (CIED)

DSVG 04 Breast implants

DSVG 05 Insulin Infusion Pumps and Integrated meter systems

16.8. Person responsible for regulatory compliance (PRRC)

Note that in accordance with Art. 15 MDR/IVDR[540], this person(s) is/are established with the appropriate qualifications, resources, procedures and responsibilities are established:

Art. 15 (3) The person responsible for regulatory compliance

shall, as a minimum, be responsible for ensuring that

...

(c) the post-market surveillance obligations in accordance with Article 10(10) (MDR; or Art. 10 (9) IVDR) are fulfilled,

d) the reporting obligations according to Articles 87 to 91 (MDR) resp. Art. 82-86 (IVDR) are fulfilled,

---

[539] https://ec.europa.eu/health/sites/health/files/md_sector/docs/md_guidance_meddevs.pdf

[540] Please see also MDCG 2019-7: Guidance on article 15 of the medical device regulation (MDR) and in vitro diagnostic device regulation (IVDR) on a 'person responsible for regulatory compliance' (PRRC)

Chapter 17. Service Part

17.1. Useful Internet addresses

Legal information systems:

https://eur-lex.europa.eu/homepage.html?locale=de
Access to European law; is a legal information system (i.e. a database of legal content) providing direct and free access to European Union legislation and other documents classified as public.

https://www.gesetze-im-internet.de/
In a joint project with juris GmbH, the Federal Ministry of Justice and Consumer Protection provides almost the entire current federal law of Germany for interested citizens free of charge on the Internet. The laws and ordinances can be called up each in their valid version.

http://www.ris.bka.gv.at/
Access to the Austrian legal information system, to consolidated legal acts and to the federal law gazettes.

https://www.admin.ch/gov/de/start/bundesrecht/systematische-sammlung.html
Systematic collection of Swiss federal law

https://de.wikipedia.org/wiki/Rechtsinformationssystem
Survey on international legal information systems, including those of EU- and EEA member states

Authorities:

EU:
https://www.camd-europe.eu/

Homepage of the competent authorities for medical devices and IVD in the EU, with interesting information on current and upcoming activities, e.g. the roadmap for the implementation of the new regulations; the FAQs on MD and IVD transitional regulations; the prioritisation of the preparation and revision of guidelines, etc.

https://ec.europa.eu/health/medical-devices-sector_en
Homepage of the Commission Services for Medical Devices with links to all essential legal and interpretative texts of the EU in the field of medical devices and IVDs, e.g. to the Medical Devices Directives and Regulations, the Guidelines (e.g. MDCG documents) of the European Union (Commission and MDCG) on Medical Devices, and reference to some older guidances to the Directives, like MEDDEVs, e.g. interpretations on the delineation of medicinal products (pharmaceuticals) and medical devices, on clinical evaluation or on the vigilance system, etc. The European Commission also displays the development of the EU's legislation and implementation, including survey of the harmonized standards, the CTS/CS, the notified bodies for the individual directives/regulations, lists of Competent Authorities and contact points in the MSs for various areas (e.g. vigilance, clinical investigation etc.); the international activities of the EU in the field of medical devices, etc.

https://ec.europa.eu/health/md_sector/new_regulations/guidance_en
Link to Guidance of the Medical Device Coordination Group (MDCG) which already addresses the new Regulations for MD and IVD; you may also find a list of forthcoming MDCG-Guidances there. MDCG-Guidances are non-legally binding documents, which interpret provisions of the Regulations. Consider them as currently best guess for interpretation.

https://ec.europa.eu/health/md_sector/current_directives_en
Access to the old guidances of the COM, esp. the MEDDEV's of the EU Commission = non-legally binding guidelines of the EU for medical devices under the Directives for all essential regulatory areas; only partly still useful for the Regulations, e.g. Vigilance, Delineation to pharmaceuticals, clinical evaluation

https://ec.europa.eu/growth/tools-databases/nando/index.cfm?fuseaction=directive.notifiedbody&dir_id=34 (NB for MDs)

https://ec.europa.eu/growth/tools-databases/nando/index.cfm?fuseaction=directive.notifiedbody&dir_id=35 (NB for IVDs)

Access to the EU **Nando** Information System to search for suitable Notified Bodies for the **MDR** and **IVDR**. You can see here the list of already designated NBs for the MDR resp. IVDR (with links to them) and pull down menues for a refined search for Annexes/Articles, product codes and codes for horizontal technical competence (see chapter XII.4. and XIII.4. in this book) to search for suitable NBs which would match your product/product portfolio

https://ec.europa.eu/health/medical-devices-sector/new-regulations/contacts_en

MD-sector contact points in the EU for:
Competent Authorities in Member States
Vigilance contact points
Clinical investigation contact points
TSE-BSE-contact points
Nando, Team-NB, NBOG, CEN, CENELEC, etc

National:
All Member States:
https://ec.europa.eu/health/md_sector/contact_en
EU national Competent Authorities contact points for:
Competent Authorities in Member States
Vigilance contact points
Clinical investigation contact points
TSE-BSE-contact points

Germany:
https://www.bundesgesundheitsministerium.de

https://www.bundesgesundheitsministerium.de/themen/gesund-heitswesen/medizinprodukte.html

Homepage of the German Health Ministry for the MD/IVD-Sector

https://www.bundesgesundheitsministerium.de/naki.html#c12535

National Working Group for the Implementation of the New EU Regulations on MD and IVD in Germany (NAKI)

https://www.bfarm.de/DE/Medizinprodukte/_node.html

Homepage of the Federal Institute for Pharmaceuticals and Medical Devices (BfArM), includes the former DIMDI German Institute for Medical Data Processing and Information with access to medical databases and medical devices

https://www.pei.de/DE/in-vitro-diagnostika/in-vitro-diagnostika-node.html

IVD-sector of the German Paul-Ehrlich-Institute

https://www.zlg.de/medizinprodukte/benennung-von-zertifizierungsstellen

Authority responsible for notified bodies, Zentralstelle der Länder für Gesundheitsschutz bei Arzneimitteln und Medizinprodukten (ZLG) with: (in German: Antworten und Beschlüsse des Erfahrungsaustauschkreises der nach dem Medizinproduktegesetz benannten Stellen (EK-Med))

Austria:

https://www.sozialministerium.at/Themen/Gesundheit/Medizin-und-Gesundheitsberufe/Medizin/Medizinprodukte.html

Homepage of the Federal Ministry of Social Affairs, Care, Health and Consumer Protection of Austria, here: Department of MD and IVD (preparation of legislation and strategic tasks)

https://www.basg.gv.at/en/medical-devices

Website of the Federal Office for Safety in Health Care and the AGES/Medical Market Surveillance for Medical Devices with access to forms for clinical investigations, free sale certificates, legislative texts etc.

Switzerland:

https://www.swissmedic.ch/swissmedic/de/home/medizinpro-dukte.html

Homepage of the Swiss Agency for Therapeutic Products, with information on the regulations for medical devices and contact details.

International:
http://www.fda.gov/MedicalDevices/default.htm
Homepage of the Center for Devices and Radiological Health of the FDA with comprehensive up-to-date information on the regulations for medical devices in the USA; information on medical devices approved in the USA; search functions; valuable guidelines for many product groups: Reports on expert panels of the CDRH

https://www.fda.gov/MedicalDevices/DeviceRegulationandGuidance/default.htm
Comprehensive range of information on US regulations for medical devices; registration in the USA, Investigational Device Exemptions (IDE), US approval procedures; guidance documents, safety information, etc.
http://www.imdrf.org/
Homepage of the International Medical Device Regulators Forum (IMDRF; successor of the Global Harmonisation Task Force - GHTF) A strategic global initiative for the harmonisation of medical device regulations; many interesting (but non-legally binding) guidelines.

Standardization:

https://ec.europa.eu/growth/single-market/european-standards/harmonised-standards/medical-devices_en
Homepage of Implementing Decisions (EU) on harmonised standards for MDR and summary list of HN
https://ec.europa.eu/growth/single-market/european-standards/harmonised-standards/iv-diagnostic-medical-devices_en
Homepage of Implementing Decisions (EU) on harmonised standards for IVDR and summary list of HN
http://www.iso.org/iso/home.html
Homepage of the International Standardization Organization (ISO) with search functions for standards
http://www.iec.ch/

Homepage of the International Electrotechnical Commission (IEC) with standards database

http://www.cen.eu/Pages/default.aspx
Homepage of the European Standardization Organization (CEN) with search functions for (e.g.) medical device standards

https://www.cenelec.eu/
Homepage of the European Standards Organisation (Cenelec) with information about (among others) medical device standards (focus: electrotechnical standards)

https://www.din.de/de
Homepage of the German Institute for Standardization (DIN)

https://www.austrian-standards.at/home/
Homepage of the Austrian Standards Institute with search functions and ordering options (also by e-mail) for standards, also for medical devices

https://www.snv.ch/
Swiss Standards Association (SNV)

Health Technology Assessment (HTA) and Evidence based Medicine (EBM):

https://www.eunethta.eu/
Network of European HTA-institutes

https://www.iqwig.de/en/
Homepage of the German Institute for Quality and Efficiency in Health Care, with numerous assessments also on medical devices and IVDs

https://aihta.at/page/homepage/en
Website of the Austrian Institute for HTA, AIHTA, (among others) with a good collection of links to Health Technology Assessments, Evidence Based Medicine and Health Economics, with a focus (also) on medical devices; numerous rapid assessments of medical devices

https://www.cochranelibrary.com/

Everything you need to know about the Cochrane library and systematic reviews; important for clinical trials; with many links to Evidence Based Medicine and Health Technology Assessment websites.

http://www.york.ac.uk/crd/
The University of York, NHS Centre for Reviews and Dissemination: Comprehensive information and link collection on Evidence Based Medicine and Health Technology Assessment with search functions

http://www.comet-initiative.org/
The COMET (Core Outcome Measures in Effectiveness Trials) Initiative brings together people interested in the development and application of agreed standardised sets of outcomes, known as 'core outcome sets' (COS). These sets represent the minimum that should be measured and reported in all clinical trials of a specific condition and are also suitable for use in clinical audit or research other than randomised trials.

Ethics Committees:

http://www.eurecnet.org/index.html
European Network of Research Ethics Committees - EUREC

https://www.ak-med-ethik-komm.de/index.php?option=com_content&view=featured&Itemid=458&lang=en
Working Group of Medical Ethics Commissions in the Federal Republic of Germany e.V.
http://www.ethikkommissionen.at/
Internet portal of the Austrian ethics committees with contact data, forms and background information
https://www.swissethics.ch/en/
Swiss Ethics Committees for Research on Human Beings

https://www.ecrin.org/

ECRIN is a public, non-profit organisation that links scientific partners and networks across Europe to facilitate multinational clinical research. ECRIN provides sponsors and investigators with advice, management services and tools to overcome hurdles to multinational trials and enhance collaboration.

Other interesting websites for medical devices:

http://www.medtecheurope.org/
Homepage of the European medical device manufacturer platform MedTechEurope with interesting information offers

https://www.bvmed.de/de/english
Website of the German Medical Technology Association BVMED
http://www.austromed.org/
The website of the Association of Austrian Medical Device Companies with comprehensive information and training opportunities

17.2. List of Figures

17.4. List of Abbreviations

AIDC	Automatic Identification and Data Capture; AIDC is a technology used to automatically capture data. AIDC technologies include bar codes, smart cards, biometrics and RFID.
AIMDD	Active Implantable Medical Device Directive = Directive 90/385/EEC
AR	Authorised Representative
Art.	Article (of MDR or IVDR)
Art. x (y)	Art. x, paragraph y of MDR or IVDR
Art. X/Y	Art. X of MDR/corresponding Art. Y of IVDR
CA	Competent Authority
CE	Conformite Europeenne, sign of compliance with EU regulations
CEAR	Clinical Evaluation Assessment Report of NB
CER	Clinical Evaluation Report (for MD) of MF
CEV	Clinical Evaluation (of MD)
CEV-Plan	Clinical Evaluation Plan
CIR	Clinical Investigation Report
CMR-ED	CMR: substances that are cancerogenic, mutagenic or reprotoxic or are suspected to have such effects; ED: Endocrine disruptors (hormonally active substances)
COM	EU-Commission
CS	Common Specification (see MDR/IVDR: Art. 9)
DA	Designating Authority for NB
Dir	Directive
EEA	European Economic Area
EP	Essential Principles, term used by GHTF/IMDRF and ISO (ISO 16142 parts 1 (for MD) and 2 (for IVD)), corresponding to Essential Requirements of previous Directives and with some differences to GSPR of new regulations
ER	Essential Requirements, previous term for requirements in Annex I, see now GSPR
GHTF	Global Harmonisation Task Force (common strategic initiative of EU, FDA, CAN, AUS and J for harmonisation of MD regulations); now superseded by IMDRF

GSPR	General Safety and Performance Requirements of Annex I of both Regulations; previous term: Essential Requirements - ER (Annex I of Directives)
HS	Harmonised European Standard
HRI	Human Readable Interpretation; HRI is a legible interpretation of the data characters encoded in the UDI carrier.
IMDRF	International Medical Device Regulatory Forum[541]: successor of GHTF, now enlarged by BR[I]CS-countries und Observers (e.g. WHO)
IMP	Importer
IVD	In-vitro Diagnostic
IVDD	In-vitro-Diagnostic Device Directive = Directive 98/79/EC
IVDR	IVD Regulation (EU) 2017/746
LC-Processes	Life Cycle Processes, e.g. QMS, Risk Management, Clinical Evaluation, Performance Evaluation, PMS, Vigilance etc.)
MDCG	Medical Device Coordination Group; acc to MDR: Art. 103 und IVDR: Art. 98
MDD	Medical Device Directive = Directive 93/42/EEC
MDSAP	Medical Device Single Audit Program of IMDRF see www.imdrf.org
MEDDEV	Medical Device Guidelines of EU-COM (non-legally binding Guidance)
MF	Manufacturer
MD	Medical Device
MDR	Medical Device Regulation (EU) 2017/745
MS	Member State of EU/EEA
NB	Notified Body (Conformity Assessment Body)
NBOG	Notified Bodies Operations Group of MS and COM
NLF	New Legislative Framework of EU for product legislation
PEAR	Performance Evaluation Assessment Report (IVD) of NB
PER	Performance Evaluation Report (IVD) of manufacturer
PEV	Performance Evaluation of IVD
PIS	Putting into Service
POM	Placing on the Market
PMCF	Post Market Clinical Follow-up (MD)

---

[541] www.imdrf.org

PMPF	Post Market Performance Follow-up (IVD)
PMS	Post-Market Surveillance
PSUR	Periodic Safety Update Report; ‚Safety Report'
QMS	Quality-Management-System
Rec	Recital (Considerations and aims of European law makers behind legal texts)
SRN	Single Registration Number (for MF, AR, IMP)
SSCP	Summary of Safety and Clinical Performance for Class III and implantable MDs (MDR: Art. 32)
SSP	Summary of Safety and Performance for IVD of Classes C+D (IVDR: Art. 29)
STD	Sexually Transmitted Diseases
subpara	Subparagraph
TSE	Transmissible Spongiform Encephalopathia; like BSE, Scrapie or CJD and vCJD
UDI	Unique Device Identifier